Pediatric Balance Program

Sieglinde Martin, M.S., PT

Illustrations by P. Jason Sauer

Therapy Skill Builders®
a division of
The Psychological Corporation

555 Academic Court
San Antonio, Texas 78204-2498
1-800-228-0752

REPRODUCING PAGES FROM THIS BOOK

As described below, some of the pages in this book may be reproduced for instructional use (not for resale). To protect your book, make a photocopy of each reproducible page. Then use that copy as a master for photocopying.

 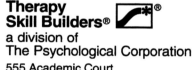

About the Author

Sieglinde Martin, M.S., PT, has been a physical therapist for 35 years, working in a variety of settings from private practice to schools to a university clinic. She developed the *Pediatric Balance Program* while working in her own private practice, Children's Physical Therapy, in Columbus, Ohio, between 1988 and 1997. She earned her physical therapy degree and licensure from the University of Cologne in Cologne, Germany, and her master's of science degree at Ohio State University in Columbus, Ohio. She also earned a fellowship in physical therapy in 1964 at the University of Kansas City, Kansas.

Ms. Martin is a member of the American Physical Therapy Association (APTA) and a member of APTA's Pediatric Section, as well as its Pediatric Study Group in Columbus. She has made presentations and published articles in journals including *Krankengymnatic, Pediatric Physical Therapy, Physical Therapy Forum,* and *Occupational Therapy Forum.*

To Allison, Amanda, Amber, Andrew, Aaron, Caleb, Camdon, Celeste, Chelsea, Christopher, Danny, Joe, Jordan, Julie, Justin, Kaily, Katie, Keith, Mary, Nick, Samantha, and Zalman

Contents

Acknowledgments

I would like to acknowledge and thank P. Jason Sauer for all the drawings. Jason graduated from Columbus College of Art and Design in May 1988. He proved his talent as an artist. His ability to understand children with disabilities and physical therapy methods is reflected in the illustrations. Thanks also go to Tanya Corzatt for taking most of the photos on which the illustrations are based, and her son Camdon for being a patient or age-appropriate impatient model for many pictures. I thank Liz Watson for her help with coordination. Thank you also, Pat Blum, for editing and correcting the text, and thanks to my husband for his help with the selection of the photos and wording.

I would like to thank all the therapists and clinical students who loved to discuss treatment strategies with me. Most of all I would like to thank my daughter Kristine, a 1989 graduate of the Ohio State University Physical Therapy Program, for listening, and offering constructive criticism, support, and encouragement.

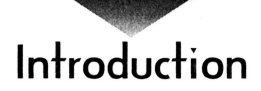

Introduction

During many years as a pediatric physical therapist, I realized the importance of balance training for children with cerebral palsy (CP). Improvement of movement and posture is not complete and does not lead to functional independence unless balance control is acquired.

Historically, it has been difficult to work on balance control with children with CP because muscle or joint contractures and spasticity did not allow for positioning in which balance training was effective. But because of many advances made in treatment and management of children with CP over the past three decades, this has changed.

Early intervention, parent involvement, neurodevelopmental treatment-based physical and occupational therapy, improved seating, positioning, and orthotics all contribute to ensuring that children with cerebral palsy maintain good joint and muscle range. Treatment and medical management of spasticity has advanced. Selective dorsal rhizotomy surgery, Botox injection, or baclofen pump implant all diminish hypertonicity permanently or temporarily. Consequently, balance exercises that were previously used only with children with mild cerebral palsy became effective for children with greater neurological involvement.

Traditionally, balance training is considered after stretching, strengthening, neuromuscular reeducation, and coordination exercises have been used. By experience, I have noted that balance training may be interwoven successfully with other treatment strategies. Balance training emphasizes unassisted, guarded activities. It establishes the foundation for independent functional activities. Consequently, early balance training promotes the earliest possible independence in various functional positions.

Balance is needed in any position where the trunk is raised off the supporting surface. Therefore, this balance program is not limited to standing balance exercises. Sitting balance with arm support is the first skill to be mastered. This manual guides you in how to increase balance demands slowly and train the child from one level to the next.

Although designed for children with cerebral palsy, the exercises and activities in this book are useful in treating children with other conditions, such as myelomeningocele and Down syndrome, as well.

HOW TO USE THE PEDIATRIC BALANCE PROGRAM

This manual is for physical or occupational therapists working with children who have cerebral palsy or balance deficits for other reasons. The exercises and activities should help pediatric therapists integrate balance training with treatment goals, strategies, service delivery, or delegation to paraprofessionals, teachers, parents, or caregivers.

The balance exercises are presented in ascending order of difficulty, with mastery of one skill being the building block for the following one. Sitting balance is addressed first. It is divided into sitting balance training with arm support, without arm support, and advanced sitting balance training. Recommendations for optimal positioning precede these chapters. Next follows balance training in four-point, kneeling, standing, squatting, and during transitions to and from standing. Crutch walking, beginning walking, as well as sidestepping and back stepping are included, with emphasis of the balance aspect of these skills. The last chapter addresses advanced balance training in terms of half standing, single leg standing, and standing on unstable ground.

The systematic presentations, clear descriptions, and illustrations should help you employ balance training effectively for all aspects of service delivery. The exercises are grouped in sets of two to six activities, which may be reproduced for therapy purposes. The illustrated exercises should be handy treatment samples when communicating treatment goals and strategies to a physical or occupational assistant. With specific instructions, they will be appropriate for a classroom or home program. For this purpose a reproducible cover sheet, "Guidelines for Balance Training," is provided. It reminds parents or teachers of basic rules to be followed and also allows space for a therapist's notes.

Each set of exercises has a common theme. Directions for positioning and preparation as well as a statement of purpose are given. Exercises have specific goals and are arranged in order of difficulty with the easiest one first. The last exercise demonstrates acquisition of the new skill. While each exercise or activity may be effectively practiced by itself, the sequential presentation will help parents or teachers. With the final goal in view, they will better understand the intent of a particular instruction and, consequently, will implement it more effectively. As the broader goal is broken down into subgoals, lay people become aware of the complexity of a seemingly easy task. This in turn, will make them more patient during practice and more appreciative of the child's efforts.

The term "activity" frequently is used instead of exercise. This is done intentionally. Its use emphasizes that treatment is merged with a simple play activity. Often, the best results are produced if the child fully concentrates on the play and not the treatment aspect of the activity.

The work of adults is subtle. They are allowed a hands-on approach only during preparation and initial practice. Balance training starts after all external support is withdrawn. Without touch, the most challenging part for child and adult begins. You, the therapist or caregiver, concentrate on and are involved in all the child's movements. You should anticipate any danger of balance loss and quickly and calmly prevent it. With vigilant eyes and ready hands to assist briefly as needed, you or another adult create a safe space in which the child experiments and learns.

Instructions for verbal guidance are given throughout the book. Supplement them as appropriate and helpful. Most of the time you will want to tell teachers or parents to direct the child verbally as little as possible and instead be responsive play partners while quietly monitoring the child's posture and movements. Play and fun are powerful self-motivators and bring better results than superfluous directions or promised rewards. When a situation does not allow play, use personal attention or an incentive (which may even be food).

Repetitions are important for new skill development Parents and teachers should be made aware of this. Even when an activity becomes easy, additional practice will be beneficial. Overlearning ensures that a skill becomes a permanent part of the child's balance repertoire. As soon as a child uses a new skill spontaneously during activities, it is established well enough to discontinue its training.

All exercises and activities should be used only under the specific direction of an occupational or physical therapist. It is at the therapist's discretion and judgment when or how to delegate them to other adults.

GUIDELINES FOR BALANCE TRAINING

1. Safety is most important. You want to make sure that your child does not get hurt during practice. Sit, kneel, or stand very close to your child and watch him or her at all times. Observe your child's posture and movement, anticipate any danger of balance loss, and quickly and calmly prevent it.
2. Guard the child with extended arms from the side or the front. Do not stand behind your child unless specified.
3. Be patient. Balance activities are much more difficult than they look. A child with poor balance has very good reasons to be afraid of falling. You want to build confidence and not frustrate the child.
4. Be calm. Create a pleasant, quiet work environment. Turn off the TV, send the dog outside, put the telephone on automatic answering, etc. You may praise your child as she does well, yet avoid boisterous cheering. Quiet, relaxed concentration helps your child to balance and gain confidence.
5. Talk to your therapist before progressing to more difficult activities. Always follow your therapist's directions.

Specific instructions for:

Name: _____

Date: _____

Therapist: _____

Sitting Balance Training

Sitting With Propped Arms

These exercises are for children who cannot sit unless they are supported by another person. Initial activities require less coordination and balance. Sometimes two or three activities of equal difficulty are presented. They train various aspects of the same skill and will contribute to better learning of the prerequisites for the more demanding later skill. Muscle tightness, joint contractures, and abnormal reflex activities of children with CP may interfere with the training of certain activities. This is addressed when appropriate.

Beginning Sitting Balance Training

These exercises are for children who sit independently with arm support. The challenge is to sit without any arm support. A quiet, relaxed situation is created that enables the child to let go of support and balance in sitting. Next, slow movements, trunk rotation, and small weight shifts are integrated.

Advanced Sitting Balance Training

These exercises are for children who are able to sit unsupported but lack the ability to stay upright when their balance is challenged or disturbed. These children may fall during play. When dressing and undressing, they rely on intermittent arm support to stay upright. Activities presented are training trunk rotation, quick postural adjustments, large weight shifts, lower extremity weight bearing, and stepping reactions.

POSITIONING FOR SITTING BALANCE TRAINING

In order to work on sitting balance, the child must be in a position that makes it physically possible to stay upright with minimal effort. The following requirements must be met:

- Center of gravity is over base of support;
- Pelvis and trunk are straight or leaning forward, and shoulders are vertically aligned with hips or in front of hips; and
- Hips and legs form a wide base of support.

The following positions fulfill these requirements and are used for balance training: sitting with propped arms, ring sitting, and bench sitting.

Sitting With Propped Arms

The child sits on floor with legs abducted, externally rotated, and flexed at the knee. The pelvis is in neutral alignment or tilted anteriorly, the trunk leans forward, and extended arms are propped for additional support. Hips, legs, and arms form a wide triangular base of support. The center of gravity is over the center of the base of support.

This is a stable position. It requires the least amount of balance. Normally developing infants sit with propped arms at 5 months of age.[1]

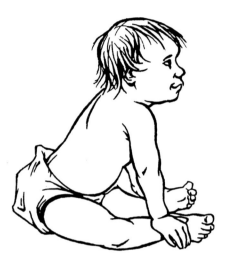

PROBLEMS WITH PROPPED SITTING

1) To maintain this position, the child must be able to bear weight over extended arms. Often children with quadriplegia cannot do this because increased flexor tone interferes with elbow extension. Arms are drawn up, and the child may be unable to voluntarily extend one or both elbows.
2) Knees are raised off the floor due to lower extremity hypertonicity. This reduces the base of support and makes the position unstable.
3) Severe hypotonia may cause arms to be too weak to support the weight of the upper trunk.

MODIFICATIONS

1) Use of Urias® pressure splints. These commercially available splints with air chambers are placed on arms. They inhibit biceps spasticity and provide reliable upper extremity support for the child with hypertonicity. For the child with weak, hypotonic muscles the splints will give stability to elbow extension. As strength or control improves, support can be reduced by inflating air chambers only partially and later by discontinuing them altogether.[2]

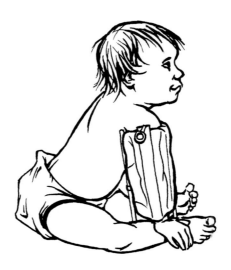

2) Use of a bench. Instead of propping the arms on the floor, the arms are propped on a low bench. This raises the trunk so that the center of gravity shifts backward and the arms bear less weight. Consequently, less arm strength or control is required to maintain the position. There is a trade-off, however. With the trunk more vertical, the center of gravity shifts posteriorly of the center of the base of support. Therefore, position becomes less stable and demands more balance control.

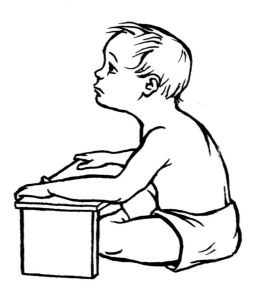

3) Use of sandbags. A sandbag is draped over each thigh. The weight of the bags will stretch adductor muscles, lower legs to the floor, and add stability to the sitting position.

Sandbags are commercially available or can be made by sewing up the legs of old jeans and filling them with sand. The size and weight of sandbags should be adjusted to the size and weight of the child. A 6″ by 12″ sandbag works well with most 2-year-old children.

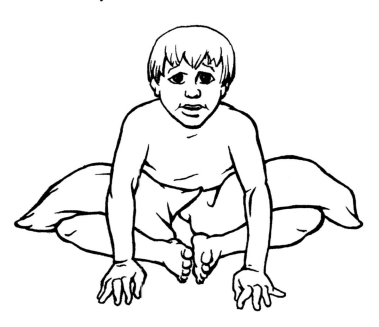

Ring Sitting

The child sits on the floor with legs abducted and externally rotated and knees flexed. The pelvis and trunk are aligned, and the arms do not bear any weight. If the child cannot keep his pelvis in a neutral position, an anterior tilt is preferable to a posterior tilt. A posterior pelvic tilt shifts center of gravity posteriorly and makes the child fall backward. As compensation, the child may round his back, which interferes with the development of a straight sitting posture.

In ring sitting, hips and legs provide a wide base of support, and the erect trunk is balanced with center of gravity positioned over the base. This is a stable position. Normally developing infants ring sit independently before they master any other sitting position without arm support. Ring sitting is safe for the beginning sitter. Loss of balance may hurt, but it usually does not cause injuries. This is the preferred treatment position when working with infants or young children.

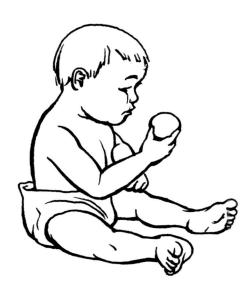

PROBLEMS WITH RING SITTING

1) Most children with diplegic cerebral palsy, and many with quadriplegia, cannot assume or maintain a ring sitting position. Because of weakness, spasticity, muscle tightness, or joint contracture, these children sit with the pelvis tilted posteriorly, a rounded back, and flexed, drawn-up legs. This is an unstable position; the base of support is narrow, the pelvis and shoulder are not aligned, and the center of gravity is posterior to the base if trunk flexors are relaxed. This unstable backward-tilted sitting position cannot be used for balance training.

2) Excessive posterior pelvic tilt reverses the action of the iliopsoas; activity of this muscle now lifts the legs off the sitting surface. When sitting with the pelvis erect or with some anterior pelvic tilt, the iliopsoas pulls the lumbar spine down and the pelvis forward as it works in synergy with the low back extensor to keep the pelvis in an optimal neutral position. For improvement of sitting balance, this muscle synergy has to be trained and mastered. Without stable legs and a fairly erect pelvis, the iliopsoas and erector spinae cannot complement each other to keep the trunk upright.

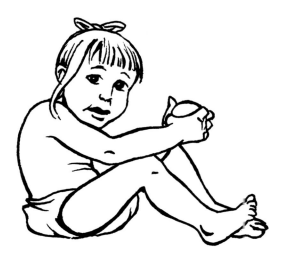

MODIFICATIONS

1) Use of a slanted or raised surface. The pelvis is lifted for passive correction of posterior pelvis tilt. A firm foam piece 1 1/2″ to 4″ thick is placed under child's hips. The thickness depends on the size of the child. A 2-year-old child may do well with a 1 1/2″ lift, while a 6-year-old may need a 4″ lift. A small Tumble Forms® wedge or a Bottoms Up seat[3] may also work well. The commercially available Bottoms Up seat is contoured to facilitate hip abduction and adds stability by enlarging the sitting surface. Having the child sit on a folded-up bath or beach towel is a simple homemade solution. For the desired effect, the hips have to be higher than the legs. When a wedge is used, the child sits in a forward-slanted position. Studies have shown that a forward-slanted sitting surface decreases posterior pelvic tilt.[4,5,6]

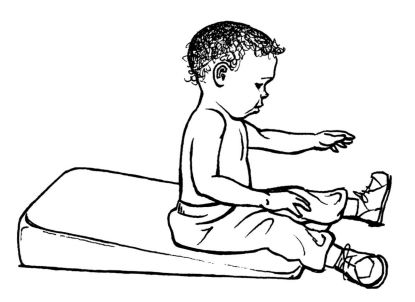

2) Use of sandbags. Even with the pelvis straight and trunk well aligned, the child with cerebral palsy may be unstable in ring sitting. Adductor hypertonicity interferes with relaxed abduction and external rotation of legs. Consequently, the legs do not rest on the floor but are drawn up and unstable. To lower the legs to the sitting surface, a sandbag is draped over each thigh. The weight of the sandbags will effect a continuous stretch to the adductors and inhibit adductor hypertonicity. Even when full range is not achieved, the weight of the sandbags may make the legs stable enough for independent sitting practice.

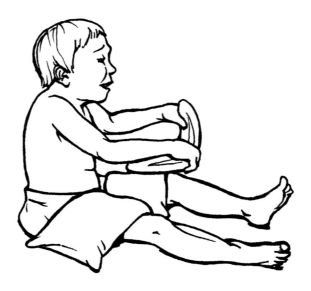

If ring sitting cannot be achieved with modification, the position cannot be used, and balance training cannot be done in ring sitting. Ring sitting with manual assistance at the hip will train trunk control but not independent sitting balance.

Bench Sitting

The child sits on the bench with his pelvis and trunk erect; hip, knees, and ankles flexed 90 degrees; and feet flat on the floor. The knees should be aligned with the hips or slightly abducted, and they should not be touching. Sitting with knees apart and feet flat on the floor increases the base of support and makes the position more stable. Bench sitting is more difficult; it requires more balance because the supporting surface is smaller than in ring sitting. Only the hips, thighs, and feet are weight bearing; yet in bench sitting it is easier to keep the pelvis in neutral alignment. This is especially true for children with CP. For this reason, a child with cerebral palsy has better balance when sitting on a bench than on the floor. Nevertheless, floor sitting is practiced first with all children because it is safer, allows independence earlier, and is age-appropriate for small children.

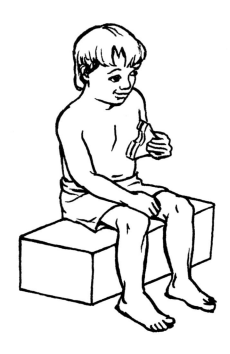

PROBLEMS WITH BENCH SITTING

1) Muscle hypertonicity may cause legs to adduct, knees to extend, and feet to plantar flex. As knees extend, the hamstrings pull the pelvis into a posterior tilt. This results in a posterior weight shift and loss of balance. Plantar flexion reduces the weight-bearing surface as the heels no longer have ground contact.

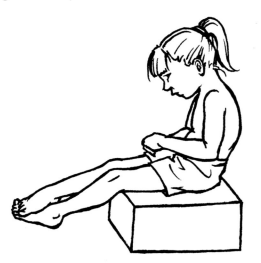

2) Bench sitting is unsafe for the beginning sitter. Loss of balance may cause serious injury. Therefore, children should not bench sit unattended until they have gained sufficient balance. Safety precautions are required for balance training in bench sitting.

MODIFICATIONS

1) Use of ankle-foot orthotics. These braces keep ankles in 90-degree flexion and allow weight bearing with the entire foot: heel, forefoot, and toes. With the ankles controlled, reflex activity diminishes, and it will be easier for the child to maintain the desired position.

2) A foam spacer placed between the thighs keeps the knees aligned and controls adductor spasticity. Commercially available pommels or abduction wedges that attach with a bracket to the underside of the sitting surface serve the same purpose.

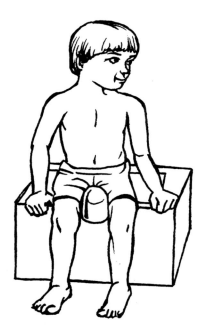

3) Use of small wedge or tilted bench.[7] The forward-tilted surface reduces posterior pelvic tilt, shifts body weight over legs, and makes legs more stable. The added stability lets the child relax and thus reduces muscle hypertonicity.

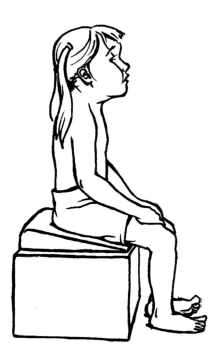

4) Use of a Nylatex[8] strap to stabilize lower extremities. Wrap 4″- or 6″-wide Nylatex strap over the child's thighs and under sitting surface. This adds stability and makes beginning bench sitting easier. As balance and control improve, use of a Nylatex strap should be discontinued.

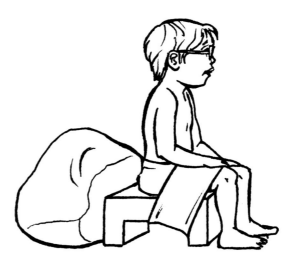

5) Use of a Kaye posture system.[9] This commercially available system is designed to keep the child's pelvis in neutral alignment, and hip, knees, and ankles at 90 degrees. It lends itself well to safe trunk balance training. As the child improves and gains control, sitting balance training should continue without the support system.

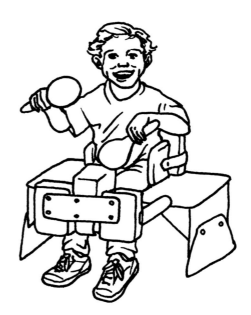

Balance Training in Sitting
With Arm Support

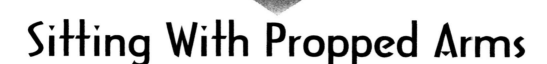

Sitting With Propped Arms

PURPOSE: Child learns to sit independently with propped arms.

PRACTICE SETUP: The child sits on the floor with her pelvis and trunk leaning forward and supported on extended arms. Her legs are placed with her knees bent and turned out. If needed, drape sandbags over the child's thighs to increase stability. As the child improves, practice without the bags.

1. Quiet sitting at a wall

The child sits with lower back against the wall. Encourage the child to lift his head and look forward. For instance, have the child watch and listen to a See 'N Say or any other interesting moving toy or display. The child may watch other children, people, pets, or a video. Discourage any movement. The quieter, the more distracted from the task, and the more relaxed the child is, the better he will do. Give intermittent assistance to legs or arms as needed. Do not give assistance to the trunk.

GOAL: The child sits for 30 seconds or longer without any assistance.

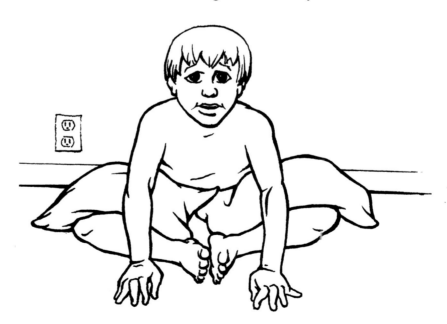

2. Sitting without back support

The child sits away from the wall with a pillow behind. Practice as in preceding activity.

GOAL: The child sits unsupported for 30 seconds or longer.

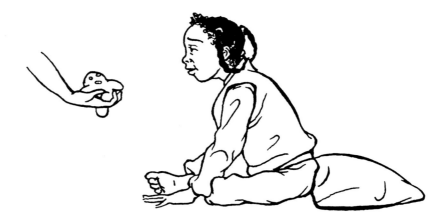

3. Sitting with side-to-side weight shift

Place your flat hands laterally on the child's shoulders and upper arms. With gentle, slow but steady pressure to the right shoulder, move the trunk to the left side until most of the upper body weight is borne by the left arm. Do the same with the other side. Do 10 weight shifts, pause, then do 10 more. Sing or play music during the activity. A steady rhythm will be helpful and will make the activity fun.

GOAL: The child will maintain balance during three sets of 10 lateral weight shifts.

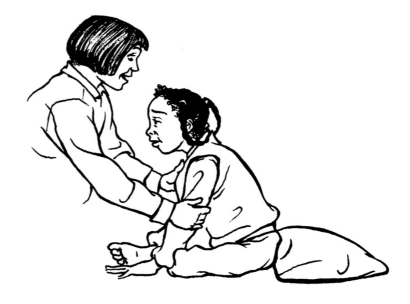

4. Sitting with head turning

Have the child look at a toy or display. Slowly move the toy to the right side and encourage the child to look all the way to the right. Slowly bring the toy back to the center and move it all the way to the left side. Repeat 10 times.

GOAL: The child keeps her balance while turning her head.

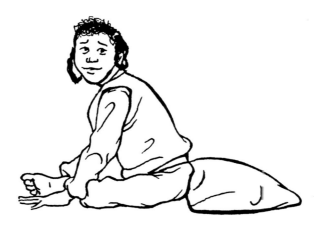

5. Sitting with brief trunk extension and guided protective extension forward

Sit in front of the child and hold her arms at or just above the elbow. Lift both arms a few inches off the floor. By doing so, the child should sit up straighter. Release your hold and encourage the child to catch herself with extended arms, wrist, and open hands. Be careful not to bring the arms up higher than the child can successfully catch herself. Do five repetitions, pause, do five more repetitions. Do more repetitions if the child is willing.

GOAL: The child develops protective extension reaction and becomes able to catch herself when losing balance.

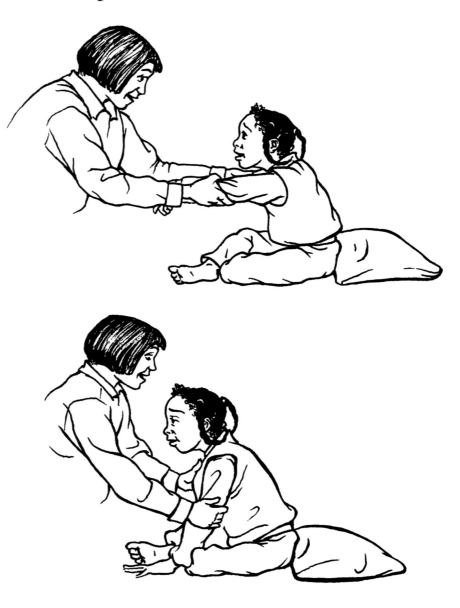

Sitting With Propped Arms and Playing

PURPOSE: The child learns to maintain a sitting position with reduced arm support.

PRACTICE SETUP: The child sits on the floor with the pelvis and trunk leaning forward and supported on extended arms. Legs are placed with knees bent and turned out. If needed, drape sandbags over the thighs to increase stability. As the child improves, practice without the bags.

1. Sitting with reach forward

Sit in front of the child. Place a simple toy in front of the child and encourage him to touch or move it. Wait for the child to initiate movement. If the child fails to do so, assist by shifting weight toward one arm while helping the child to lift the other arm. Practice with either arm.

GOAL: The child will lift either hand while supporting himself with the other hand. The child will do simple play activities in sitting.

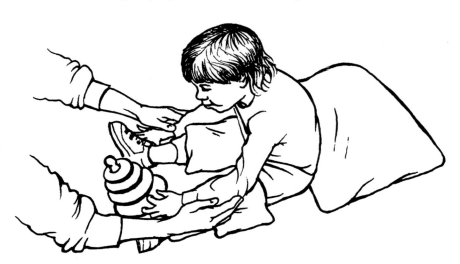

2. Sitting with reach up

Sit in front of the child. Hold up an interesting toy and encourage the child to reach up with one hand while supporting himself with the other hand. Practice with either hand.

GOAL: The child props himself on one hand while reaching up and playing with the other hand.

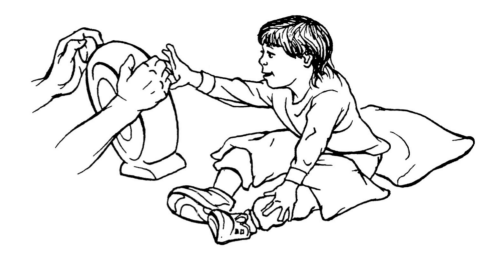

3. Independent sitting with play

As the child gains enough balance and control to sit with propped arms, provide plenty of practice opportunities. Place a favorite toy in front and encourage the child to play independently. Initially, the child may do best with his low back against a support and sandbags draped over his thighs.

GOAL: The child sits independently with propped arms and plays for 10 minutes or longer.

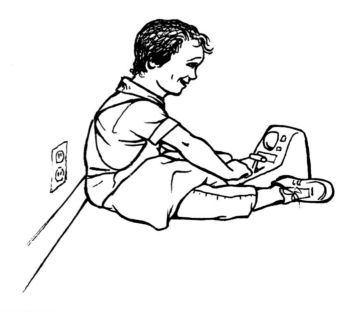

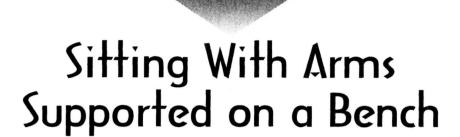

Sitting With Arms Supported on a Bench

PURPOSE: The child learns to balance in floor-sitting while leaning with his arms on a bench.

PRACTICE SETUP: The child sits on the floor in front of a low bench. The child's legs are folded Indian style or placed with knees bent and turned out. Her pelvis and trunk lean forward and arms rest on the bench. A lap tray is a good substitute for a bench. Practice on a carpeted floor or mat, and place a pillow behind the child.

1. Quiet sitting with hands on a bench

Sit in front of the child. Place the child's open hands on the bench and put your hands on top of them. Talk to the child and encourage him to look at you. Have the child concentrate on your words, sounds, and facial expressions; discourage any movements. Slowly withdraw your hands and start counting aloud as long as the child stays seated. Do three to 10 repetitions, depending on the child's tolerance.

GOAL: The child sits with hands on a bench for 30 seconds without any assistance.

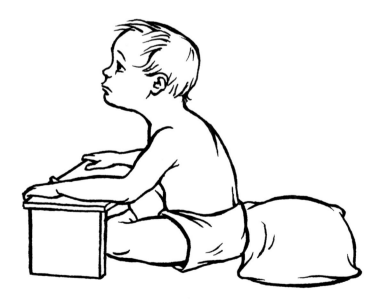

2. Sitting with one hand on a bench

Sit in front of the child. Place a simple toy, such as a roly poly chicken or other simple toy, on the bench and encourage the child to play with one hand while steadying himself with the other hand or forearm. Initially, assist by placing your hand over the child's supporting hand. Withdraw your support as the child improves. Have the child play with either hand.

GOAL: The child plays for 1 minute while supporting himself with one hand on bench and playing with other hand.

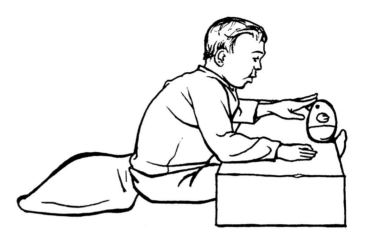

3. Sitting with one hand on a bench

Practice as in the preceding activity. Play with the child and encourage him to reach up high or slightly to the side. Assist by steadying the child's supporting arm if needed. Encourage play with either hand.

GOAL: The child sits with one arm supported on a bench and reaches with the other arm.

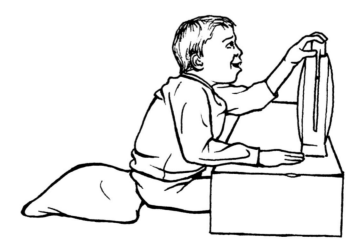

4. Independent sitting with play at a bench

After the child has gained enough balance and control to sit with arms propped at a bench, provide plenty of opportunities to practice this skill. Place a favorite toy on the bench and encourage the child to play independently.

GOAL: The child plays at a bench for several minutes without any assistance.

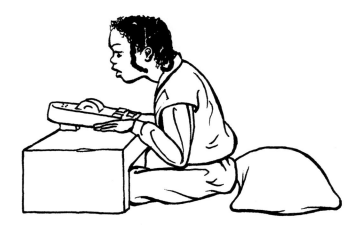

Sitting Holding Onto a Stick

PURPOSE: Exercises train beginning sitting balance. Weight shift and trunk rotation are introduced.

PRACTICE SETUP: The child sits on the floor with his pelvis and trunk straight. The child's legs are folded Indian style or placed with knees bent and turned out. If needed, drape sandbags over his thighs to increase stability. As the child improves, practice without bags. Practice on a carpeted floor or on a mat and place a pillow behind the child.

1. Quiet sitting holding onto a stick

Sit facing the child with your legs stretched out so the child sits between your legs. Help the child to grasp the bar. Place your hands over the child's if they slip off. Talk to the child and encourage him to look at you. Have the child concentrate on your words, sounds, and facial expressions; discourage any movements. As the child pays attention and balances, intermittently take your hands off and let the child hold onto the stick independently. Do three to 10 repetitions, depending on tolerance.

GOAL: The child sits independently holding onto a stick with both hands for brief time periods.

2. Sitting holding onto a stick

Sit facing the child with your legs stretched out so the child sits between your legs. Present a horizontal stick and ask the child to hold onto it. If needed, assist by lightly placing your hands over the child's. Encourage the child to lean forward and hold on tight. Slowly move your hands to side and:

a) count to 5, 10, 15, or as long as the child holds on and sits;
b) sing a song or recite a nursery rhyme to make the activity fun for the child.

GOAL: The child sits holding onto a stick for 30 seconds or longer.

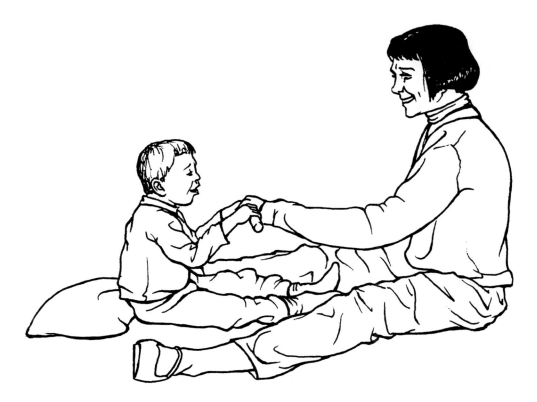

3. Sitting holding onto a stick with weight shift

Start practicing as in the preceding activity. Once the child holds onto the stick well, sing with child and:

a) slowly move the stick up and down;
b) slowly move the stick to the right side and then to the left side.

Monitor the child's posture. Discourage the child from slouching backward into a posterior pelvic tilt.

GOAL: The child sits and shifts weight forward, backward, and side-to-side while holding onto a stick.

4. Sitting, holding onto a stick, with trunk rotation

Start practicing as in the preceding activities. Once the child holds onto the stick well, play music or sing and slowly move the stick all the way to the right side and then to the left side. Encourage the child to rotate shoulders and look to the side. Move with the rhythm and do numerous repetitions. Monitor the child's posture. Discourage the child from slouching backward into a posterior pelvic tilt.

GOAL: The child sits and rotates trunk while holding onto the stick.

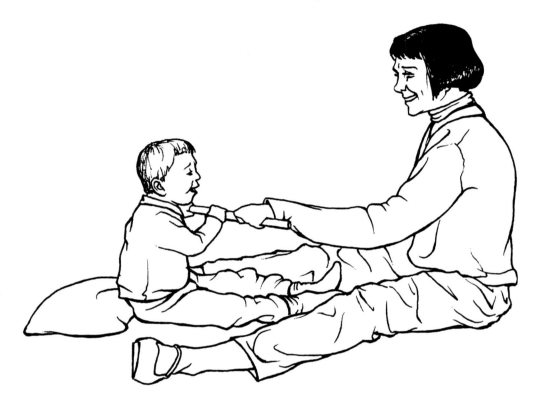

Bench Sitting Holding Onto a Bar

PURPOSE: Activities train beginning sitting balance. The child learns to sit independently on a bench or chair while holding onto a bar.

PRACTICE SETUP: The child sits on a bench with her trunk straight and leaning slightly forward. Her hips, knees, and ankles are flexed 90 degrees, and her feet are flat on the floor. Her knees should be aligned with her hips and not touching. This will ensure a wide base of support and decrease influence of abnormal reflex of lower extremities. Have the child sit in front of a ladder[10] or ladderbox.[11]

1. Bench sitting holding onto a ladder with both hands

Ask the child to hold onto a rung of a ladder with both hands. If the child cannot do this, assist from the side or front by placing your hands over the child's. Tell her to hold on tight. Slowly withdraw your hands and

a) count aloud to 5, 10, 15, or as long as the child holds on and sits independently;
b) sing a song or recite a nursery rhyme while the child sits independently.

As the child improves, ask her to straighten elbows and sit as tall as possible.

GOAL: The child sits independently, holding onto a rung of a ladder for 30 seconds or longer.

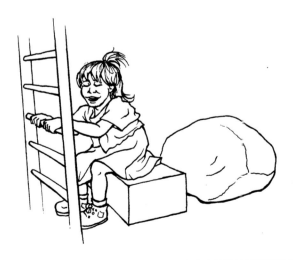

2. Bench sitting with variable arm support

The child holds onto the rung of a ladder with both hands. Ask the child to take his right hand off the rung, reach up, and hold onto a higher rung. Repeat with the left hand. Next ask the child to move his hands back down, one hand at a time. Do several repetitions. Closely guard and remind the child not to take both hands off simultaneously but always to hold on with one hand.

GOAL: The child sits independently, holding onto a rung of a ladder with one or both hands.

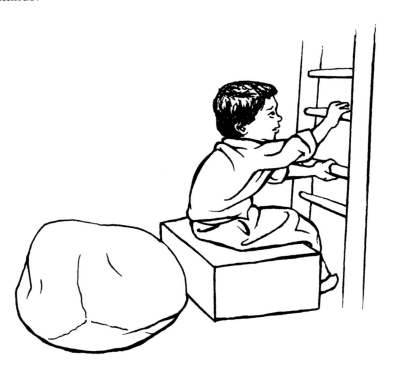

3. Bench sitting with variable arm support and play

These activities are similar to the preceding ones but include a play element that enhances participation.

a) Drape a beanbag animal over the rung two places higher than the starting rung. Encourage the child to release one hand from a rung, move it up, push the animal down, and then hold onto the rung again. Do many repetitions and practice with either hand. As a challenge, place the beanbag on increasingly higher or lower rungs. For variety, hang a string of beads, ribbons, or other suitable items over rungs. A stuffed animal may be squeezed between rungs and the child asked to "rescue" it.

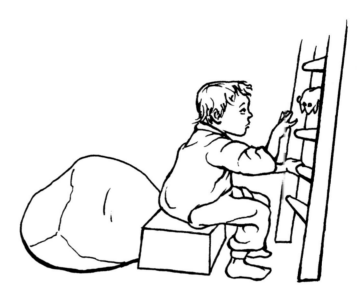

b) Place an upright bolster to the right side. Encourage the child to move his right hand off the rung and push the bolster down. The child will enjoy the thumping noise as the bolster drops to the floor. After the child has returned his right hand and securely holds onto the rung, place the bolster to the left side and repeat the activity. Have a stuffed animal perched on the bolster for more fun.

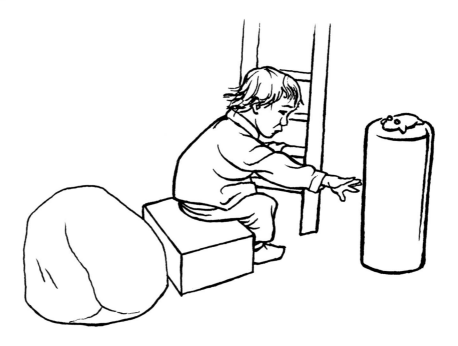

GOAL: The child sits independently holding onto a rung of a ladder with one or two hands.

4. Bench sitting with one-hand support and trunk movement

The child holds onto a rung of the ladder with both hands. Drop a beanbag next to the child's right foot. Ask him to pick it up and hand it to you. Do numerous repetitions and practice on either side. This activity can be combined easily with Activity 3a.

GOAL: The child sits, holds on with one hand, and moves trunk without loss of balance.

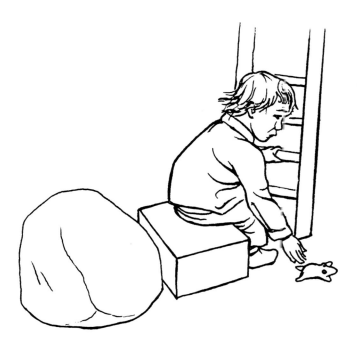

Bench Sitting at a Table

PURPOSE: The child learns to sit at the table without loss of balance.

PRACTICE SETUP: The child sits at a chest-high table. Her trunk leans forward slightly, and both elbows rest on the table. Her hips, knees, and ankles are flexed 90 degrees, and her feet are flat on the floor. Place a large beanbag chair behind the child.

1. Sitting at a table with bilateral arm support

Lead the child in a quiet activity. Looking at a picture book, doing an easy puzzle, or manipulating a tape player and listening to music will relax the child and keep her attention while sitting without external support.

GOAL: The child sits independently at a table during quiet play.

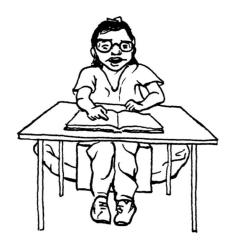

2. Sitting with variable arm support

Lead the child in an activity that requires lifting one elbow off the table (e.g., the child eats a cracker, turns pages of a book, stacks blocks or rings).

GOAL: The child sits independently at a table doing a variety of activities.

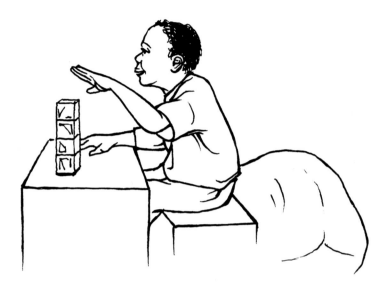

Sitting Balance Training

Beginning Floor Sitting

PURPOSE: The child learns to rise to a sitting position and maintains it for a short time without any arm support.

PRACTICE SETUP: The child sits on the floor with knees bent and turned out. Her trunk leans forward and is supported by extended arms. If needed, drape sandbags over her thighs to increase stability. As the child improves, practice without bags. Have the child sit on a raised or slanted surface to correct a posterior pelvic tilt. Sit in front of the child and place a large pillow behind her.

1. Sitting up with and without arm support

Hold a See 'N Say or other toy in front of the child and tell her to "come up and hear what the farmer says." Encourage child to:

a) come up and play holding onto the toy;

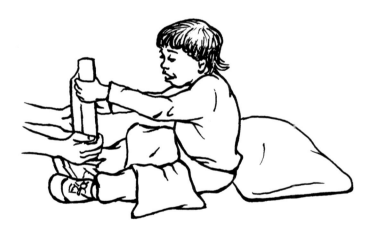

b) come up and play intermittently holding onto the toy;

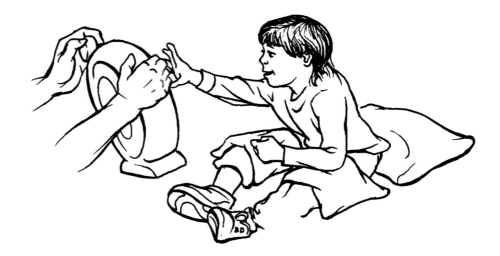

c) come up and stay up without holding on.

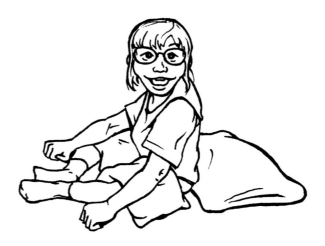

Repeat as long as the child is interested.

GOAL: The child sits up and maintains the position for brief time periods.

2. Sitting without arm support

Present two cymbals, pom-poms, or other two-handed toys and encourage the child to grasp one with each hand. Have the child clap them together and play as long as possible.

GOAL: The child sits independently while playing in midline with both hands.

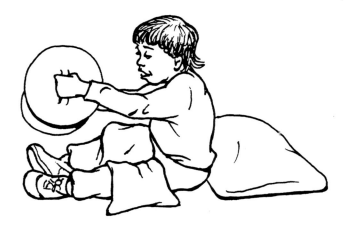

Protected Floor Sitting With Play

PURPOSE: The child learns to sit independently and play without arm support.

PRACTICE SETUP: The child sits on the floor with her pelvis and trunk straight or leaning slightly forward. Her legs are placed with knees bent and turned out. If needed:

a) have the child sit on a raised or slanted surface to correct a posterior pelvic tilt;
b) drape sandbags over thighs to increase stability.

ACTIVITY: Sit with your legs stretched out and apart. Have the child sit between your legs, facing you. Place a toy in front of the child and encourage play with both hands. First, brace the child with your legs. As the child gains balance, move your legs a few inches away and challenge the child to sit and play independently. Monitor the child closely and be prepared to give intermittent support if needed.

GOAL: Protected from falling to the side, the child sits and plays independently for increasingly longer time periods.

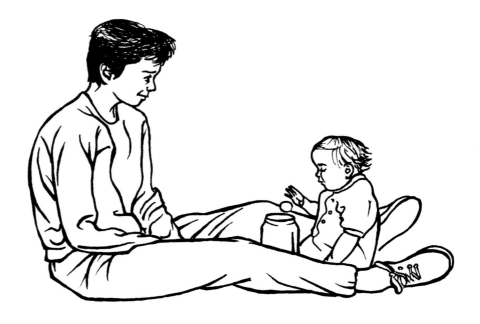

Floor Sitting With Weight Shift and Reach

PURPOSE: The child learns to shift weight and use arms in sitting without a loss of balance.

PRACTICE SETUP: The child sits on the floor with pelvis and trunk straight or leaning slightly forward. Legs are placed with knees bent and turned out. If needed:

a) have the child sit on a raised or slanted surface to correct a posterior pelvic tilt;

b) drape sandbags over thighs to increase stability.

Place a large pillow behind the child. Kneel or sit in front of the child.

1. Sitting with small weight shifts

Hold a See 'N Say or other attractive toy in front of the child. Encourage him to look and listen while you slowly move the toy up and down or from side to side. Do this as long as the child is interested.

GOAL: The child sits independently during forward and backward and side-to-side weight shift.

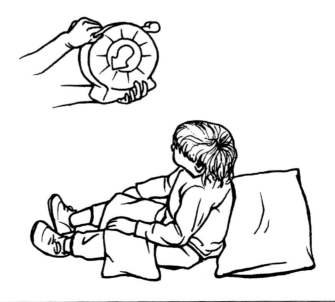

2. Reaching with one arm

Play with the child and encourage him to reach forward and to the side. First, hold a toy at easy reach, and then progress to far reach. Practice with either hand. If the child loses his balance, encourage him to catch himself with his outstretched arm. Do numerous repetitions.

GOAL: The child sits and reaches with one hand without a loss of balance.

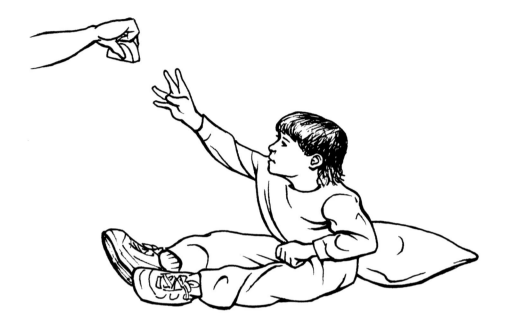

3. Reaching with both hands

Play with the child as in the preceding activity. This time, ask the child to reach up with both hands for a token. Do numerous repetitions.

GOAL: The child sits and reaches with both hands without a loss of balance.

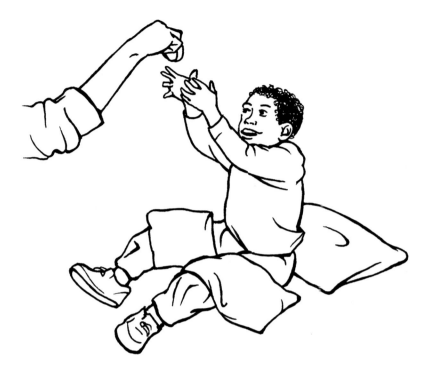

4. Playing ball

Roll a ball to the child and encourage the child to roll the ball back to you. Roll the ball slowly, using a 6″ or larger ball. You want the child to be successful, to enjoy the game, and to play as long as possible.

GOAL: The child receives and rolls a ball without a loss of balance.

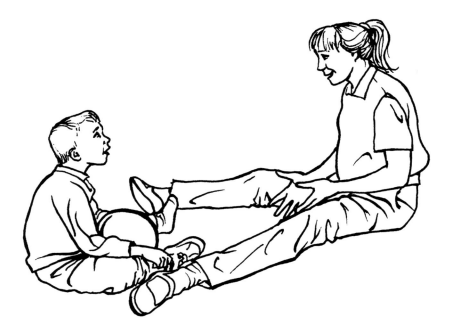

Beginning Bench Sitting

PURPOSE: The child learns to sit independently for short time periods.

PRACTICE SETUP: Sit or kneel in front of the child. Assist and support the child in sitting on a bench with her pelvis and trunk straight or leaning slightly forward. Her hips, knees, and ankles should be flexed 90 degrees, and feet flat on the floor. Her knees should be aligned with hips and not touching. If necessary, practice first with and later without a:

a) pommel, abduction wedge, or piece of foam to keep knees apart;
b) Nylatex strap to stabilize thighs;
c) wedge or tilted bench to correct posterior pelvic tilt.

Put a large pillow behind the bench or place the bench in front of upholstered furniture.

1. Quiet independent sitting

Help the child brace her trunk with her arms by placing her hands either on the bench or on her thighs. Put your hands over the child's, assisting her to steady herself. Talk to the child and encourage her to look at you. Have the child concentrate on your words, sounds, and facial expressions; discourage any movements. As the child gains balance, withdraw your hand and present a favorite picture book or other interesting display. Hold it in front, encouraging the child to look, listen and talk to you.

GOAL: The child sits independently, with quiet attention, for 30 seconds or longer.

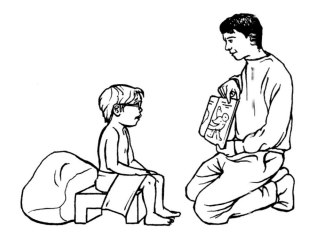

2. Protected sitting with play

Sit with legs stretched out and apart. Have the child sit on a bench between your legs, facing you. Ask the child to sit tall, bracing herself with her arms on her thighs. As the child gains balance, present a toy closely in front. Encourage the child to play with one hand while steadying herself with the other hand. Intermittently assist as needed by placing your hand over the child's. Have the child play with either hand.

GOAL: The child sits for several minutes playing with one hand while steadying herself with the other hand.

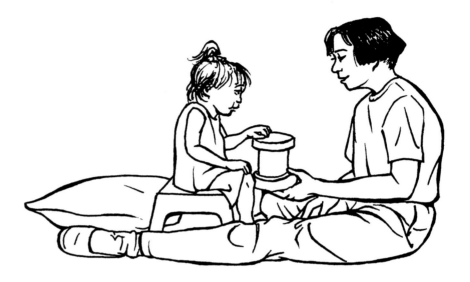

3. Sitting with one hand movement

The child sits and balances with her hands placed on her thighs. Encourage the child to eat cookie pieces while sitting without support. First, place a piece into the child's hand. Later, have the child reach forward to grasp it. Practice with either hand. Sitting quietly is a tedious task for most children. Allowing a child to eat a favorite food makes it rewarding and fun.

GOAL: The child sits independently for several minutes.

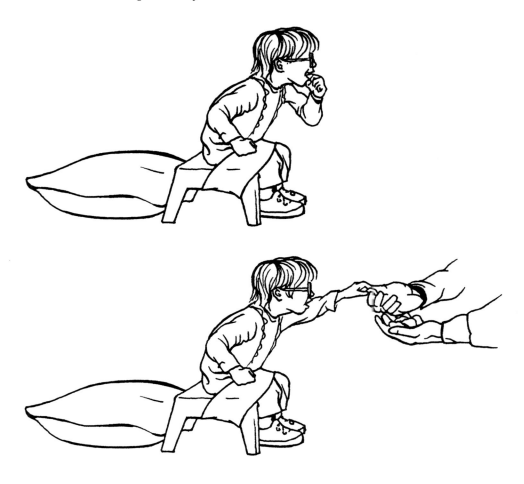

4. Independent sitting with two-hand play

The child sits and balances with his hands placed on his thighs or on the bench. Present a pop bead close to his right hand and encourage the child to grasp it. Next present a bead close to the child's left hand and have him grasp the bead. Encourage the child to push the beads together. Do numerous repetitions as long as the child is interested.

GOAL: The child sits independently without any arm support.

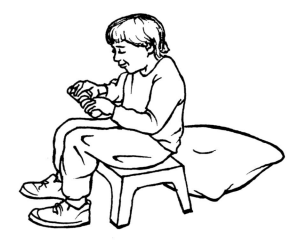

Bench Sitting With Reach and Play

PURPOSE: This activity trains beginning sitting balance. Weight shift and trunk rotation are introduced.

PRACTICE SETUP: The child sits on a bench with his trunk straight, feet flat on the floor, knees aligned with hips, and knees not touching. Put a large pillow behind the bench or place the bench in front of upholstered furniture.

ACTIVITY: Be in front and play with the child.

a) Have the child reach up.

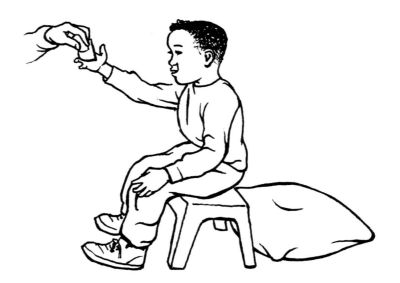

b) Have the child reach down.

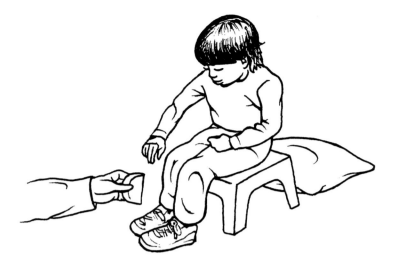

c) Encourage the child to reach to either side and to turn to the side.

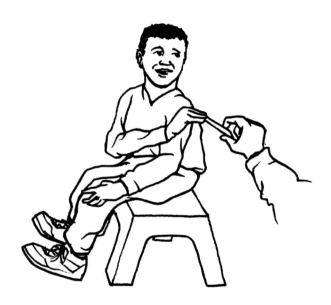

Practice with either hand or both hands. Monitor the child's posture and remind the child not to press his knees together. Do not ask the child to reach farther than he is able to. You want to build confidence, not test limits. Play as long as the child is interested.

GOAL: The child sits independently, moves trunk, shifts weight, and turns without a loss of balance.

Advanced Sitting Balance Training

Training of Quick Postural Adjustments in Floor Sitting

PURPOSE: The child learns to counteract when balance is challenged.

PRACTICE SETUP: The child sits on a mat or carpeted floor with his pelvis and trunk straight. His legs are folded Indian style or placed with his knees bent and turned out. His arms do not bear weight.

1. Sitting challenged by mild pushes

Tell the child to sit tall and be strong. Say to him, "Do not let me push you down!" Give mild pushes with your open hand to the child's trunk—to the sides, forward, backward, and diagonally. Start with slow pushes, increase pressure, and do quick taps. Adjust pressure to the child's ability to withstand it. You want to challenge the child without causing a loss of balance. Do three sets of 10 pushes.

GOAL: The child makes quick postural adjustments to pushes in all directions.

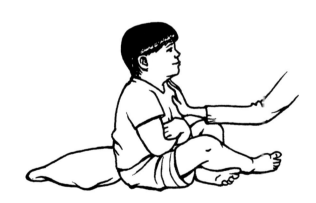

2. Paddle ball play in sitting

Hang a Wiffle™ ball from the ceiling at an appropriate height. Give the child a lightweight paddle and encourage him to play tether ball. A Boom Paddle will work well. Children enjoy the sound of a successful hit and become motivated to play (work) as hard and as long as they possibly can.

GOAL: The child makes quick postural adjustments in all directions and uses trunk rotation without a loss of sitting balance.

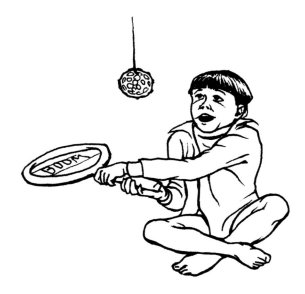

3. Ball play in sitting

Encourage the child to play ball with you. Catching as well as throwing will challenge his balance. Use balls of different sizes and weight in accordance with the child's ability. A light, medium-size ball will be easier to catch and toss than a large, heavy one. Small balls are difficult to catch but fun to throw. Roll a ball to the child if he cannot catch the ball. Play as long as the child is interested.

GOAL: The child controls quick anterior and posterior weight shifts without loss of balance.

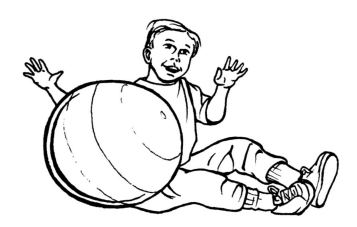

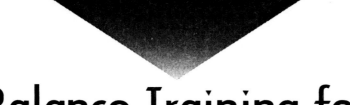

Balance Training for Functional Skills

PURPOSE: The child acquires the balance needed for dressing and grooming.

PRACTICE SETUP: The child sits on a mat or carpeted floor with his pelvis and trunk straight. His legs are folded Indian style or placed with his knees bent and turned out.

1. Reaching far

Challenge the child to reach as far and as high as possible. Use the child's favorite stacking rings or entice with a snack such as cookie pieces. Wait to give the child a reward until he stretches, shifts weight, and stretches more. Practice with either hand or both hands at the same time, reaching in all directions. Play as long as the child is interested.

GOAL: The child reaches and stretches without a loss of balance, a prerequisite for self-dressing.

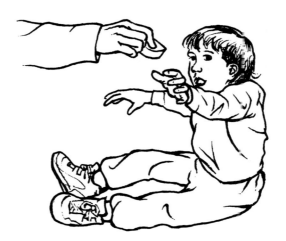

2. Donning and doffing a hat

Collect five different hats or caps. (A diaper or piece of cloth will also do.) Place one item on the child's head, and let the child look at herself in a mirror. Wait for the child's reaction. Most likely the child will reach up and pull the head gear down. After examining it, the child may try to put it back on. Encourage all play with the hat. As the child loses interest, place a different hat on her head. Continue until the child has tried all five hats or as long as she is interested.

GOAL: The child learns to manipulate with both hands overhead without a loss of balance. This is a prerequisite for pulling on a shirt or sweaters, or grooming hair.

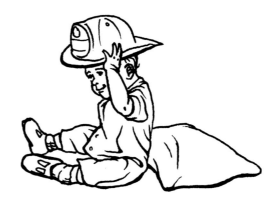

3. Donning and doffing a necklace

Collect five strings of beads or sturdy necklaces of various sizes. Put a necklace on the child, and let her look at herself in a mirror. Wait for the child's reaction. Most likely the child will get hold of the necklace, try to pull it over her head, look at it, and try to put it on again. Encourage all play with the necklace. As the child loses interest, present another necklace. Continue until the child has tried all five necklaces or as long as she is interested.

GOAL: The child learns to pull something over her head without a loss of balance. This skill is a prerequisite for pulling a shirt or sweater on or off.

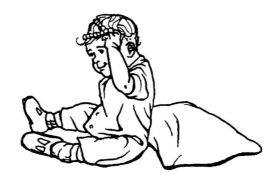

4. Pulling off and putting on socks

Gather five socks of various sizes and thicknesses. Pull one sock over the child's toes and forefoot. Wait for her reaction. Most likely the child will reach forward and pull the sock off. After examining it, the child may try to put the sock back on. Encourage all hand and foot play. As the child gets bored, place a different sock on her other foot. Continue until the child has played with all socks or as long as she is interested.

GOAL: The child combines forward and downward weight shift with movements of all extremities without a loss of balance. The child successfully takes off and pulls on socks.

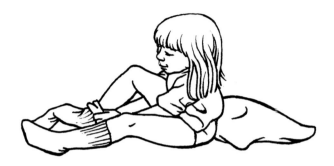

5. Pulling off and putting on footwear

Gather five different footwear items—shoes, slippers, boots, etc.—of proper fitting or somewhat larger size. Put a shoe on the child's foot without tying the laces. Encourage the child to lift and draw up his foot in order to pull off the shoe. The child may want to roll backward; do not allow him to take the shoe off while lying back. Challenge the child to take the different footwear items off either foot while sitting independently.

GOAL: The child maintains sitting balance while lifting either foot. The child successfully takes off shoes.

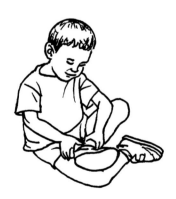

Training of Quick Postural Adjustments in Bench Sitting

PURPOSE: The child learns to counteract when balance is challenged.

PRACTICE SETUP: The child sits on a bench with his trunk straight, feet flat on the floor, knees aligned with hips, and knees not touching. Place the bench in front of upholstered furniture or place a large beanbag behind the bench. Sit or kneel across from the child.

1. Sitting challenged by mild pushes

Tell the child to fold his arms across his chest, to sit tall, and be strong. Say to the child, "Do not let me push you down!" Give mild pushes with your open hand to the child's trunk—to the sides, forward, backward, and diagonally. Start with slow pushes, increase pressure, and do quick taps. Adjust pressure to the child's ability to withstand it. You want to challenge the child without causing a loss of balance. Do three sets of 10 pushes.

GOAL: The child makes quick postural adjustments to small pushes in all directions.

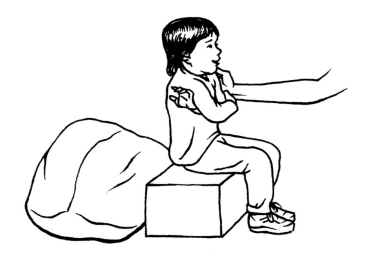

---

2. Balloon toss in sitting

Encourage the child to toss a balloon with you. Always toss the balloon into the easiest range. You do not want to make the game any harder, but reinforce success. Monitor the child's posture. Tell the child not to lean backward, but forward, as the toss is made. Play as long as the child is interested.

GOAL: The child initiates quick weight shifts and makes postural adjustments without a loss of balance.

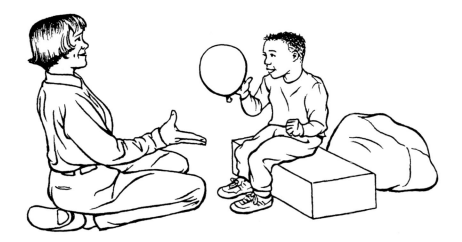

3. Tether balloon in sitting

Hang a balloon from the ceiling at appropriate height and encourage the child to toss the balloon again and again, using either or both hands. Cheer the child on, saying "Hit the balloon as hard as you can!" Monitor the child closely, and be ready to assist if he loses balance. Ask the child to "fix" posture if necessary. Play as long as the child is interested.

GOAL: The child initiates quick postural adjustments without a loss of balance.

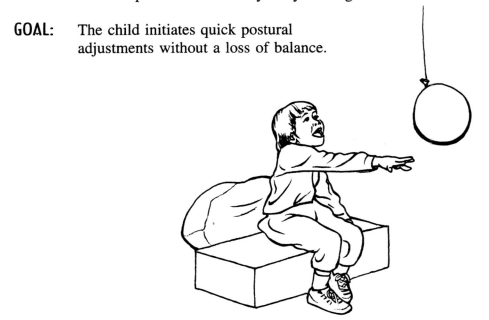

4. Ball play in sitting

Choose a lightweight, medium-size ball and encourage the child to play ball with you. Monitor the child closely. Tell the child to lean forward as he catches or throws the ball. Play as long as the child is interested.

GOAL: The child responds appropriately as balance is challenged.

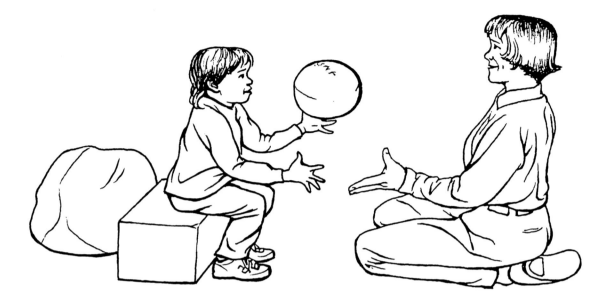

Advanced Balance Training in Bench Sitting

PURPOSE: This activity trains large weight shifts in all directions, controlled movements, and trunk rotation in bench sitting without loss of balance. The child is challenged to expand reach and balance control.

PRACTICE SETUP: The child sits on a bench with his trunk straight, feet flat on the floor. His knees are aligned with his hips and not touching. Place the bench in front of upholstered furniture or place a large beanbag chair behind the bench. Sit or kneel across from the child.

1. Far reach with play

Make reaching high, far, and turning part of a favorite game. For instance, as the child plays with a jukebox, slowly move it farther away, enticing him to lean far forward and reach for a token. Or challenge the child to toss a beanbag into a basket. Hold the beanbag in front, to the side, or sideways and backward. Give the child time to reach, weight shift, stretch, and finally pull the beanbag out of your hand. Challenge the child's limits without frustrating him or her. Practice with either hand and have the child turn to either side.

GOAL: Without loss of balance, the child weight shifts far, reaches, and turns.

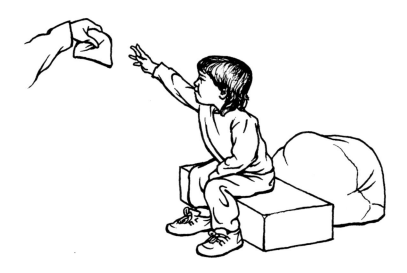

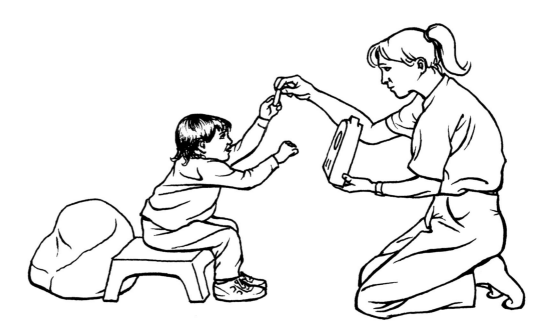

2. Reaching far with both arms

Hold up a large, light item, like a hoop, and challenge the child to stretch, reach, stretch some more, and finally get hold of the hoop. Hold the hoop forward, high, and to the sides, and encourage trunk rotation. Work slowly. You do not want to frustrate the child but gradually expand limits.

GOAL: Without a loss of balance, the child shifts weight far, reaches with both arms, and turns trunk.

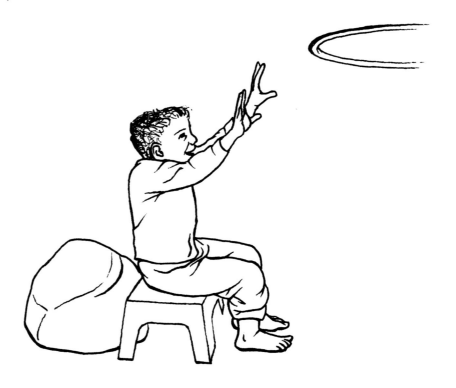

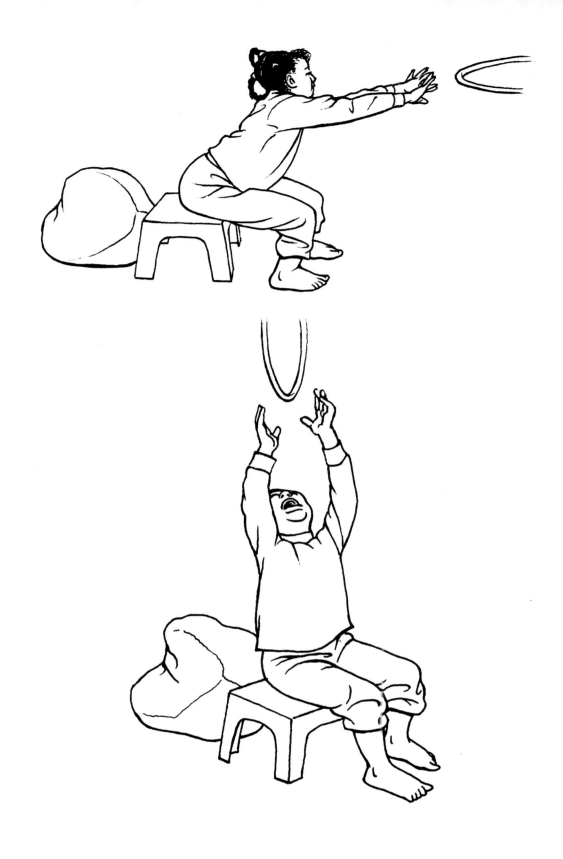

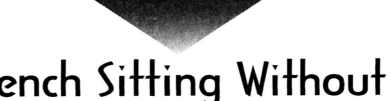

Bench Sitting Without Ground Contact

PURPOSE: Training of trunk control and balance without relying on feet for support.

COMMENT: In everyday life situations, schoolchildren are frequently required to sit on benches or chairs too high for their feet to touch the floor. While this should be avoided if a child has poor sitting balance, it may not always be possible. For instance, a mainstreamed child with cerebral palsy may want to eat with his or her classmates in the school cafeteria. Sitting without ground contact is far more difficult than sitting with feet on the floor. Make the child aware of this and give him or her time to adjust and balance. Carefully grade activities.

PRACTICE SETUP: The child sits on a bench with trunk straight. Hips and knees are flexed 90 degrees, and feet are off the ground. Sit facing the child and be ready to assist if the child loses balance. For safety reasons, place the bench in front of upholstered furniture or place a large beanbag behind the bench.

1. Balancing with reach

After the child is comfortable on a high bench, have him practice reaching for pop beads or other toys. Start in close range and gradually have the child reach farther. Monitor the child; make the activity simpler if he shows signs of stress or fear. You want to build confidence, not test limits.

GOAL: The child maintains sitting balance while reaching.

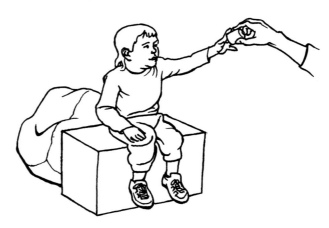

2. Balance training for functional activities

Pretend to be having a picnic. Hand the child a make-believe sandwich to unwrap and munch on. Have him drink some water, lick a pretend ice cream cone, and so on. Closely watch the child and assist as needed.

GOAL: The child sits confidently on a high bench.

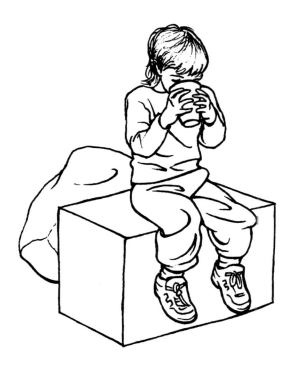

3. Moving sideways

Ask the child to place his hands at his sides on the bench and scoot to side, as if making room for another person to sit down. Model the activity, telling the child to lean on his right arm while scooting to the left. Practice moving to either side.

GOAL: The child maintains sitting balance while scooting to the side.

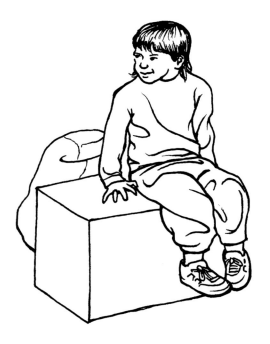

4. Moving feet

Ask the child to place his hands at his sides on the bench. Hold up
a balloon and encourage the child to kick it. Do not cheer the child on.
The child should kick only as hard as possible without a loss of balance.
Practice kicking with either foot.

GOAL: The child maintains balance while kicking.

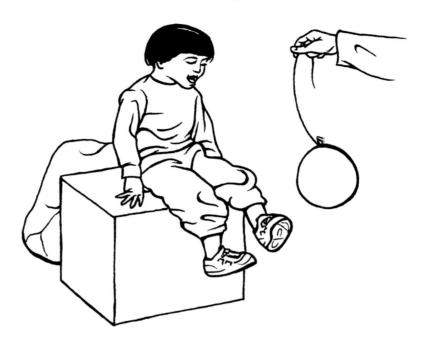

Training of Weight Bearing With Feet During Bench Sitting

PURPOSE: The following activities and exercises reinforce weight bearing over feet in bench sitting. Optimal weight bearing over feet increases a child's base of support, reinforces good posture, and improves sitting balance.

PRACTICE SETUP: The child sits on a bench with feet flat on the floor, knees aligned with hips, and knees not touching. Sit across from the child or guard at his side.

1. Pressing down with one foot

Place a small dog toy or other squeaker under the child's foot. Encourage the child to push down and make the toy squeak. If unsuccessful, tell the child to lean forward and press down on his knee with his hands. Ask the child to squeak the toy 10 times with each foot, first with arms assisting, and later without.

GOAL: The child learns to bear down with either foot.

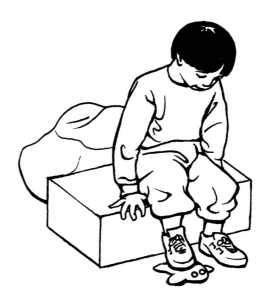

2. Foot tug-of-war

Place a towel, newspaper, or sheet of paper under the child's feet and tell him, "Press down as hard as you can. Do not let me pull it away!" Tug on the towel, encouraging the child to work hard pushing feet down. Monitor the child's posture. Remind him not to press his knees together or turn his feet in. Play five times each with the towel, newspaper and sheet of paper.

GOAL: The child learns to press down with both feet.

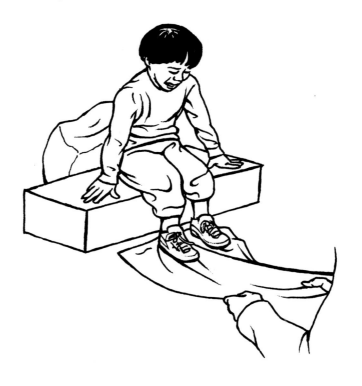

3. Play with low forward reach

Create a play situation during which the child has to reach and lean down and forward. This will effect a strong forward weight shift and reinforce weight bearing over feet. Sample activities are:

a) Leaning forward and dressing up a stuffed toy;

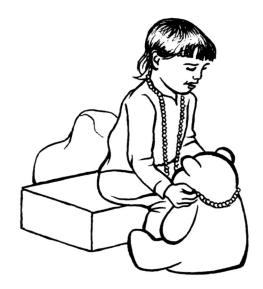

b) Reaching for a toy on the floor; and

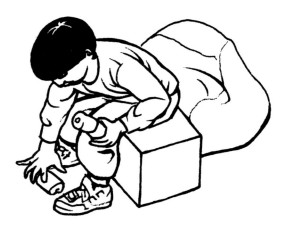

c) Reaching with a grabber.

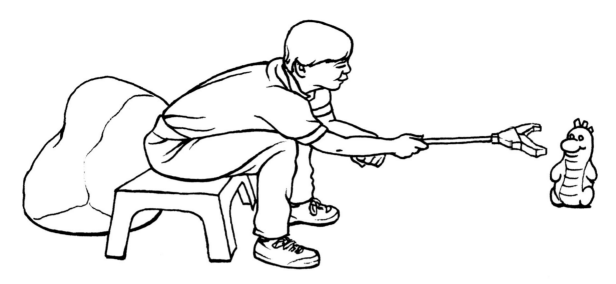

4. Thera-Band® pull

Tie a Thera-Band® in loops at ends or use an exerciser. Place one loop under the child's foot and have the child hold the other end with his hand. Tell the child to be strong and pull the Thera-Band or exerciser as far as possible. Have the child exercise five to 10 times with either foot.

GOAL: The child pushes feet down against resistance.

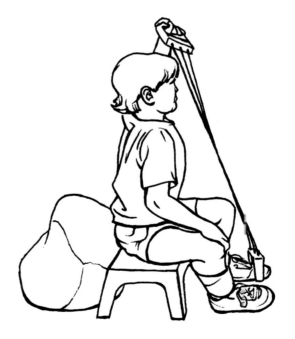

5. Lifting hand weights

Give the child a 1/2-pound weight in each hand. Encourage him to exercise like the "big guys." Have the child do arm curls, horizontal extensions, abductions, or overhead lifts with both arms at the same time. Encourage several repetitions with good form—straight trunk, chin tucked, shoulders depressed, and movement through full range of motion.

GOAL: The child bears weight over feet and shows good trunk posture during arm exercises in sitting.

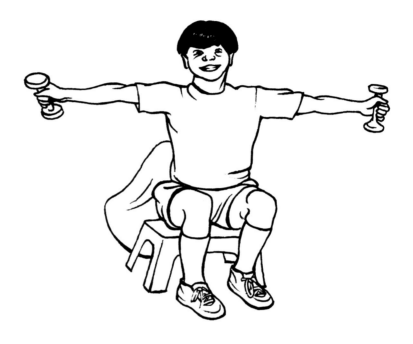

Sitting Balance Training
With a Physio-Ball

PURPOSE: The child becomes aware of boundaries of sitting balance and is challenged to expand them.

PRACTICE SETUP: The child sits on a mobile surface with her feet flat on the floor and her knees aligned with her hips. Guard the child well from the side. A Tumble Forms roll, Physio-Roll™, Physio-Ball, or T-stool may be used with the Tumble Forms roll being the most stable sitting surface and the T-stool being the least stable. Many therapists prefer the inflated Physio-Roll or Physio-Ball because the ball's bounciness adds dynamic and gentle joint compression.

ACTIVITIES: Hold the ball and help the child sit down on it. Support her at the hips or hold hands. Encourage her to balance independently. Withdraw your support as soon as the child is comfortable. Guard her well from the side. Encourage the child to:

a) Sit quietly on the ball for count of 10;

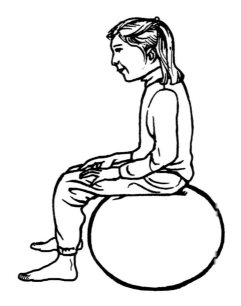

---

b) Do small side-to-side weight shifts;

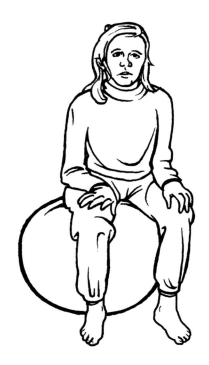

c) Clap hands together;

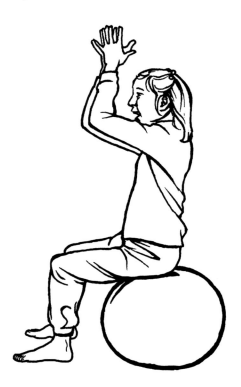

d) Bounce gently up and down;

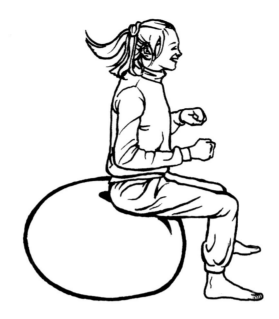

e) Swing pom-poms alternately at sides and overhead (play music);

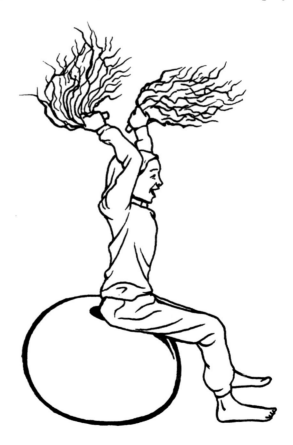

Sitting Balance Training With a Physio-Ball   **77**

f) Move legs up and down, one at a time, or march in place;

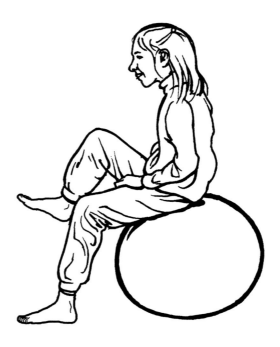

g) Straighten legs, one at a time; and

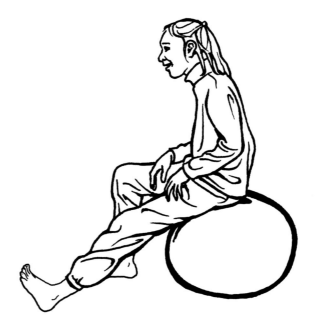

h) Move one leg out to side and do large sideways weight shifts.

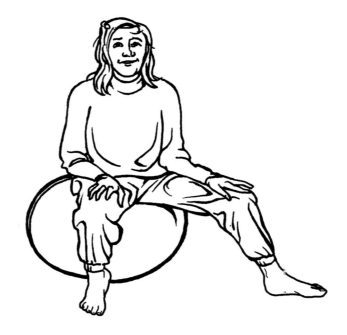

Sitting Balance Training on a Mobile Surface

PURPOSE: The child becomes aware of boundaries of sitting balance and is challenged to expand them.

PRACTICE SETUP: The child tailor or ring sits on a mobile surface. A balance board or platform swing may be used, with the balance board being safer and the platform swing more challenging and fun for the older child.

1. Induced weight shifts on a balance board

The child sits on a balance board with arms at sides. Tell her: "Sit tall, do not fall down! Let's pretend you are in a boat and big waves are coming!" Slowly tip the board from side to side, forward and backward, and then randomly in any direction. Increase the speed and amplitude of motion as long as the child can tolerate it. You want to challenge the child without causing a loss of balance. Keeping her arms at her sides will allow the child to use protective extension reaction to catch herself in case of balance loss.

GOAL: The child makes postural adjustments to weight shift in all directions.

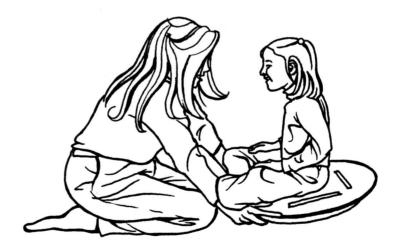

2. Independent sitting on a balance board with weight shift

First, encourage the child to sit still and balance on board. Next, ask her to make the board tip from side to side, forward and backward, or in all directions. Watch the child closely and assist as needed.

GOAL: The child balances independently and shifts weight.

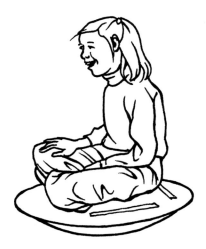

3. Induced weight shift on a platform swing

The child sits on a platform swing. Tell her: "Sit tall! Let's pretend you are flying on a magic carpet!" Slowly swing the child from side to side, forward and backward, or have the swing go around in a circle. Watch her carefully at all times to detect any unsteadiness or potential loss of balance and to prevent a fall.

GOAL: The child makes postural adjustments to weight shifts in all directions.

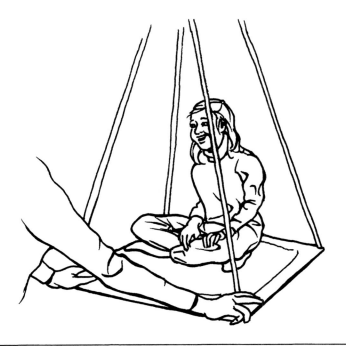

4. Independent sitting with reach on a platform swing

The child sits quietly on a platform swing without arm support. Have her reach for toys in all directions. Have the child do an easy reach first, and then challenge her to stretch and reach. The platform swing will accentuate anticipatory weight shift and force the child to carefully fine-tune all movements.

GOAL: The child learns slow, controlled weight shifts while balance is challenged.

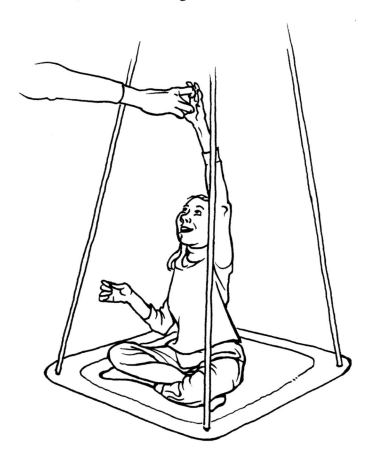

Balance Training in Four-Point

PURPOSE: The child learns to maintain a four-point position. Weight shift and balance—prerequisites for crawling on hands and knees—are trained.

PRACTICE SETUP: Practice on a soft carpet, blanket, or Airex mat.[12]

1. Quiet four-point position with hips over heels

Place the child on hands and knees with hip flexion greater than 90 degrees. Most of the weight is borne over the lower extremities. Assist at the upper arms and elbows if necessary. As the child successfully bears weight over extended arms, reduce your support. Brace the child's hips at the sides and slowly withdraw support as the child gains control. Have the child watch a music box or other display as long as the child remains in four-point position. Encourage the child to look forward.

GOAL: The child maintains a modified four-point position for 30 seconds or longer.

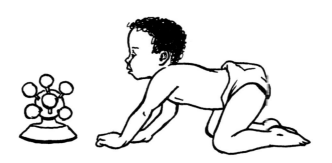

2. Four-point position with forward weight shift

Place the child on his hands and knees with hip flexion greater than 90 degrees. Most of the weight is borne over the lower extremities. Play music; support the child's hips and gently rock him forward and backward. First move the child just a couple of inches forward and then back. Increase movement until the child's weight is borne equally over hands and knees. Encourage the child to rock with music, unassisted.

GOAL: The child rocks in four-point position and becomes able to bear weight equally over hands and knees.

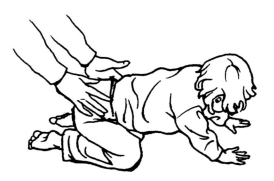

3. Play in four-point position

Place the child in four-point position in front of a pop-up box or other enticing toy. Brace his right elbow as you gently shift weight over his right arm. Encourage the child to reach and play with his left hand. Withdraw your support as soon as he shows an ability to bear weight with his right arm. Repeat the activity, having the child support his weight with his left arm and play with his right arm.

GOAL: The child becomes able to play in four-point position.

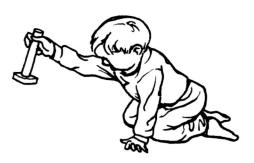

4. Advanced four-point balance practice on mobile surface

Hold a rocking board or platform swing still, and tell the child to crawl onto the center of the mobile surface. Guard her as you slowly let go of the mobile surface. Have the child balance and rock while you give standby assistance. You can upgrade the exercise by tipping the balance board in all directions or by gently swinging or spinning platform swing.

PRECAUTION: This exercise is not suitable for children under 4 years of age. Older diplegic or hemiplegic children may enjoy the challenge. You may want the child to wear a protective helmet for safety reasons.

GOAL: The child learns advanced balance skills in four-point position.

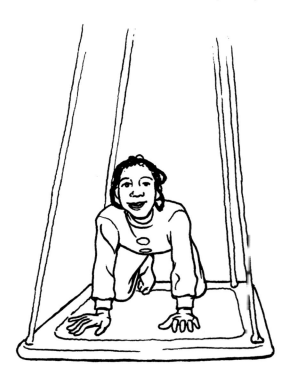

Balance Training in Kneeling

Kneeling With Arm Support

PURPOSE: The child moves into and out of kneeling and maintains the position with upper extremity support. Activities progress in difficulty. During the first activity, the child supports himself with his trunk and elbows. Later, the child is challenged to balance in kneeling with minimal hand support.

PRACTICE SETUP: Place the child in a heel-sitting or four-point position in front of stable furniture of appropriate size—chest high or a little lower. Guard the child from the right or left side. Do not give back support.

1. Quiet kneeling with upper extremity support

Encourage the child to pull himself to a kneeling position at the furniture; assist as needed. Have the child look at an attractive display or book while kneeling. Monitor posture and correct it as needed. Hips should be straight and in alignment with shoulders. You may first allow and later discourage the child from leaning with his trunk against the support. Facilitate controlled lowering to heel-sit as the child gets tired or loses balance.

GOAL: The child kneels at furniture and moves into and out of position with control.

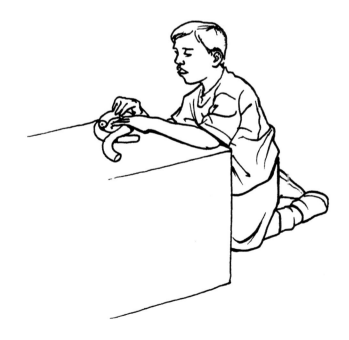

2. Kneeling with variable upper extremity support

Present a favorite toy in easy reach. Encourage the child to pull to a kneeling position and play with one or both hands. Guard the child from the side and discourage him from leaning with his trunk against the support. Facilitate controlled lowering to heel-sit as the child gets tired or loses balance.

GOAL: The child plays while kneeling with variable arm support for 1 minute or longer.

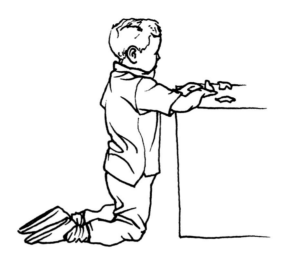

3. Independent kneeling with upper extremity support

As the child's balance and control in kneeling improve, entice him to play independently in this position.

a) Place interesting items in a chest-high drawer opened part way. Clip clothespins at the sides so the drawer will not accidentally shut and pinch the child's fingers.
b) Have the child play at a heavy, large toy box.
c) Place a large cardboard box upside down and use it as a play table for the child.

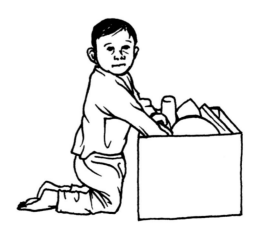

4. Kneeling at a wall

Encourage the child to heel-sit and rise to a kneeling position at a wall. Give assistance as needed. To encourage play in kneeling, mount a blackboard, felt board, cork board, or picture on the wall at an appropriate height. Other ideas are:

• Play with Colorforms® at a large mirror.
• Play with shaving cream at a glass patio door. (Cleaning up afterward with a wet sponge will be lots of fun and more exercise.)
• Play with magnets at the refrigerator.

GOAL: Bracing with hands against flat surface, the child plays while kneeling for several minutes.

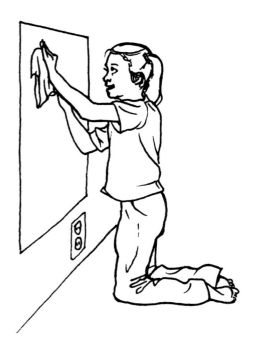

Weight Shift and Stepping in Kneeling With Arm Support

PURPOSE: The child learns to shift weight and briefly support weight over one knee. The strategy of controlled falls to the sides is introduced. Mastery will facilitate similar activities in standing.

PRACTICE SETUP: The child kneels at a stable piece of furniture of an appropriate size—chest high or a little lower. Assist the child from behind during initial practice. As the child improves, give intermittent or standby assistance from the side or front.

1. Weight shift in kneeling with upper extremity support

The child plays while kneeling at the furniture. Move a toy to the right or left side and encourage a weight shift as the child reaches for the toy. Initially assist weight shift by moving his pelvis to the side and supporting it during reach. Reduce and fade support as the child improves. If the child loses his balance to the side, facilitate sliding into side-sit and breaking the fall with an outstretched arm.

GOAL: The child learns controlled weight shifts with a reach to either side and a controlled fall to the side with a loss of balance.

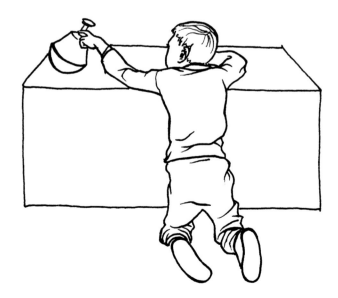

2. Sidestepping on knees with upper extremity support

The child plays while kneeling at the furniture. Place a toy to the side out of reach and encourage the child to sidestep and retrieve it. Assist by shifting weight over the left hip as the child lifts his right leg and sidesteps to the right. Assist the weight shift toward his right hip as the child steps with his left leg. Reduce and fade support as the child gains control. If the child loses his balance to the side, facilitate lowering into side-sit and breaking the fall with an outstretched arm.

GOAL: The child independently sidesteps on knees and holds onto furniture for balance support. The child falls to the side with control.

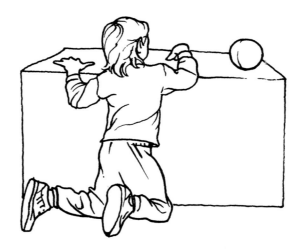

3. Sidestepping along a wall while kneeling

The child kneels at a wall, mirror, glass door, or other flat surface. Entice him to sidestep to a picture, sticker, or other object on the wall a few feet away. If needed, help him by supporting his weight-bearing leg and assisting his step to the side. As the child gains control, fade your support.

GOAL: The child independently sidesteps along the wall.

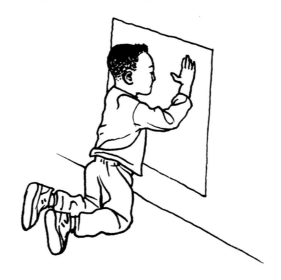

4. Forward stepping on knees with upper extremity support

The child kneels at a chest-high cardboard box, stool, or walking toy. Support the child at the pelvis and assist weight shift and full weight bearing·over one knee and stepping with other knee as the child kneelwalks, pushing a toy cart, box, or stool. Reduce and fade your support as the child gains control.

GOAL: The child independently kneelwalks, pushing a box, stool, or toy.

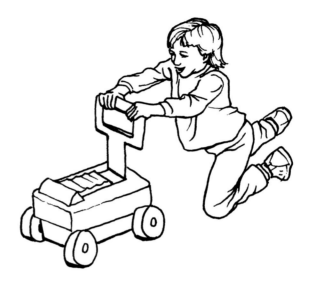

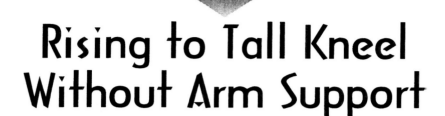

Rising to Tall Kneel Without Arm Support

PURPOSE: Activities train coordination and balance as required for raising the trunk from heel-sitting to tall kneeling.

PRACTICE SETUP: Practice on an Airex mat or carpeted floor away from furniture.

1. Rising to kneel with minimal arm support

Have the child heel-sit facing you. Hold up a container and encourage the child to come look and reach into it. Help the child with your free hand at the hip. Do 10 or more repetitions. Motivate the child by placing an interesting new toy in the container. Withdraw your support as the child improves.

GOAL: The child raises to tall kneel with minimal one hand support.

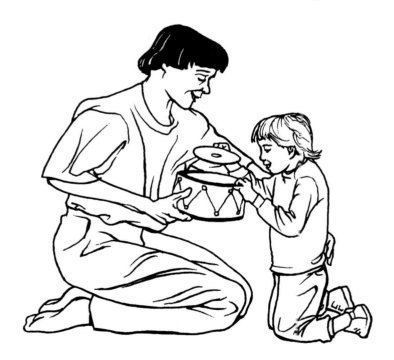

2. Rising to kneel without arm support

Place a drumstick in each of the child's hands and hold up a drum. Encourage the child to come and play the drum. If needed, help the child at the hip to rise up and guard him while he plays the drum independently. Do as many repetitions as possible. Hold up a different drum or box to beat on as an extra incentive.

GOAL: The child rises to tall kneel without holding on with his arms.

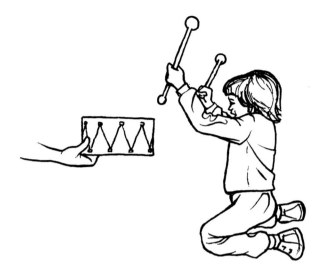

3. Rising to kneel without arm support

Hang a trapeze bar overhead. Encourage the child to rise up, reach for the bar, and swing from it. Start out by having the bar within easy reach. As the child improves, raise the bar to ensure that he comes up as tall as possible. Most children enjoy the activity and work hard, reaching up again and again to get hold of the bar and swing.

GOAL: The child rises to tall kneel without any support.

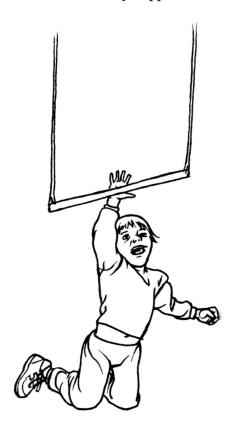

Kneeling Without Arm Support

PURPOSE: Activities train trunk control, posture, and balance required for independent standing. Training is safer and less demanding than standing balance training.

PRACTICE SETUP: Practice on an Airex mat or carpeted floor away from any furniture.

1. Quiet kneeling without support

Ask the child to kneel and hold both hands open in front. As soon as the child manages to assume the position, reward him by dropping beads or some other surprise into his hands. As the child succeeds, encourage him to stay up longer by counting to two, three, four, five, or longer before dropping a reward into his hands.

GOAL: The child balances while kneeling for 10 seconds or longer.

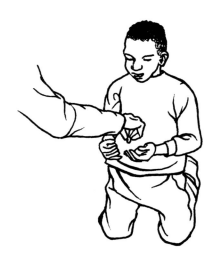

2. Kneeling with some bilateral arm movements

As the child's balance in kneeling improves, encourage him to play while kneeling. Playing a drum or cymbals can be fun and challenging.

GOAL: The child plays in kneeling for 30 seconds or longer.

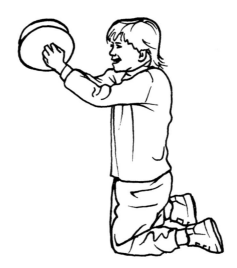

3. Kneeling challenged by mild pushes

Tell the child to kneel tall and be strong. Say to the child, "Do not let me push you down!" Give the child mild pushes with open hand to her trunk—to the sides, forward, backward, and diagonally. Start with slow pushes, increase pressure, and do quick taps. You want to challenge the child without causing a loss of balance. Do three sets of pushes.

GOAL: The child makes quick postural adjustments to an induced weight shift and improves balance in tall kneeling.

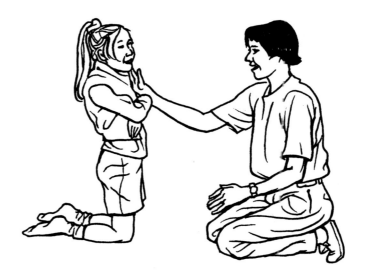

4. Ball play in kneeling

Catching as well as throwing will challenge a child's balance. Use balls of different sizes and weights according to the child's ability. A light, medium-size ball will be easier to catch and toss than a large, heavy ball. Small balls are too difficult to catch but fun to throw.

GOAL: The child plays ball for several minutes without a loss of balance.

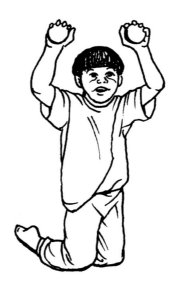

5. Lifting Tumble Forms roll in kneeling

Playing "weightlifting" is fun, especially for little boys. Holding or lifting a Tumble Forms roll will tax their strength as well as their balance. Small hand weights of 1/2 or 1 pound may also be used. The child may show better trunk extension and postural alignment with weightlifting.

GOAL: The child will show good postural alignment and balance in tall kneeling.

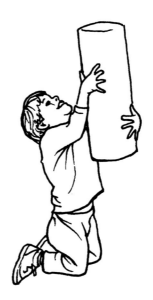

6. Kneeling on a mobile surface

Have the child kneel on a balance board. Ask her to balance for 10, 20, or 30 counts.

GOAL: The child kneels on a balance board for 30 seconds or longer.

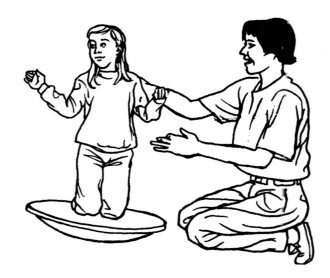

7. Advanced balance training on a mobile surface

The child kneels on a balance board. Slowly tip the board side to side, forward and backward, or diagonally. Encourage him to kneel tall and balance.

GOAL: The child successfully adjusts posture when tipped in any direction.

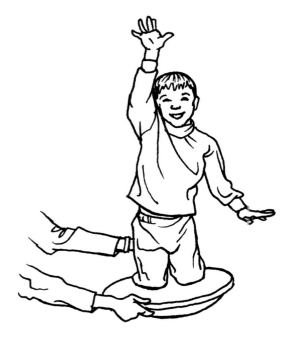

Kneelwalking

PURPOSE: Kneelwalking requires trunk control, weight shift, and balance similar to walking. Independent kneelwalking prepares children for independent walking.

PRACTICE SETUP: The child kneels on an Airex exercise mat or carpeted floor.

1. Kneelwalking in parallel bars

Place parallel bars in the lowest setting and encourage the child to kneelwalk between the bars, lightly holding on. Challenge him to place only one finger or an open hand on the bars. Also have the child try to hold on with just one hand.

GOAL: The child kneelwalks between parallel bars with minimal support.

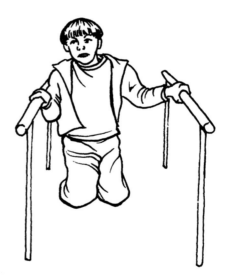

2. Kneelwalking with sticks or rings

Hold a short stick or a ring in each hand and encourage the child to hold on to them. Ask him to kneelwalk with you, holding onto the stick for balance support. As the child improves, intermittently release your grasp of the stick, encouraging the child to kneelwalk without support. Initially, be behind the child. As the child improves, be in front of him during practice.

GOAL: The child kneelwalks with minimal support.

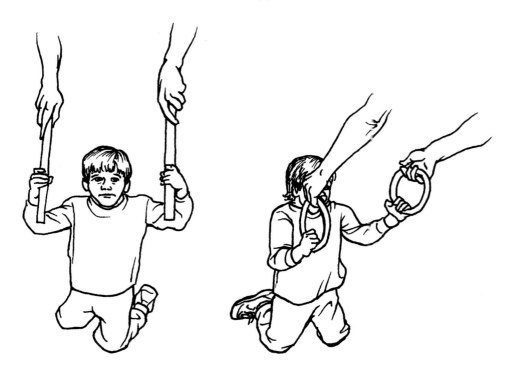

3. Independent kneelwalking

Hand the child two stuffed or soft toys and kneel 2 feet away. Encourage the child to come to you by saying, "Bring me the hippos!" (Holding stuffed toys encourages the child to stay upright and move forward without pushing off the floor with hands.)

GOAL: The child kneelwalks several steps without a loss of balance.

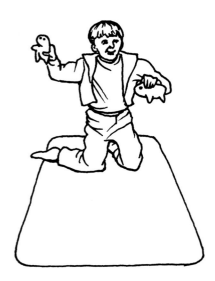

4. Kneelwalking with trunk control

Place a little water in a plastic cup, hand it to the child, and challenge him to carry it to a place several feet away. Tell him "Piggy is thirsty. Bring her some water. Move slowly so it won't spill!"

GOAL: The child kneelwalks slowly without excessive lateral or sagittal movements.

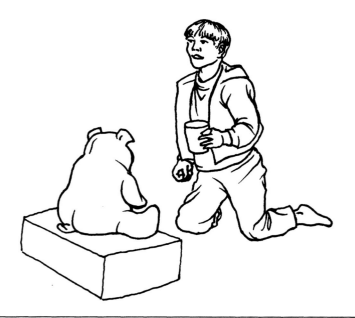

Half-Kneeling With Minimal or No Support

PURPOSE: Half-kneeling trains unilateral weight bearing over the kneeling leg. It requires more hip and trunk control than kneeling. Half-kneel is difficult for children with cerebral palsy. Pre-walking children with cerebral palsy usually require maximum or moderate support in a half-kneel. Consequently, half-kneeling cannot be used for balance training. The following activities are for walking children with mild cerebral palsy or children with poor balance for other reasons.

PRACTICE SETUP: The child kneels on an Airex mat or carpeted floor, away from furniture. Sit or kneel in front of the child.

1. Half-kneel with minimal assistance

Ask the child to half-kneel. Assist by applying downward pressure with your hand to the child's flexed knee. Encourage a straight trunk and hips and arms stretched to the sides. Challenge the child to maintain good posture and balance while counting to 10, 20, 30, or 50. Fade and withdraw your support as the child gains control.

GOAL: The child maintains good posture and balance unassisted for increasingly longer time periods.

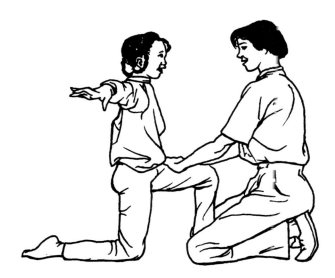

2. Half-kneel with arm movements

Give pom-poms to the child, play music, and encourage her to swing pom-poms and do cheers in half-kneel.

GOAL: The child half-kneels, with good posture and arm movements, for 1 minute.

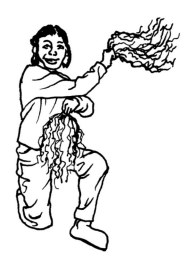

3. Half-kneel with play and reach

Play beanbag toss with the child. Present a beanbag high on the child's kneeling side and have her reach for it with her same side hand. Encourage light tosses at a specific target or into a basket. The child plays with her right or left leg forward.

GOAL: The child half-kneels and reaches high with her arm on the kneeling side without a loss of balance. (The activity is challenging because it makes the kneeling leg do most of the weight bearing.)

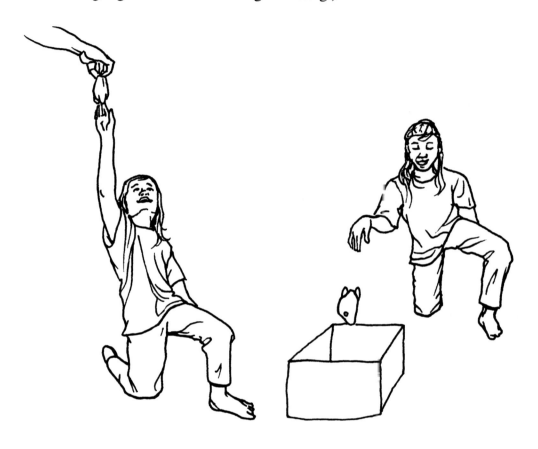

Beginning Standing Balance Training

Standing Balance Training

BEGINNING STANDING BALANCE TRAINING

These exercises are for children who cannot stand or walk unless supported by another person. Step by step the child learns to stand first with arm support, then with reduced support, and finally with no support. Acquisition of independent standing balance is a slow and complex process. Beginning exercises act as building blocks for later skills. These subskills should be trained until mastered with ease and confidence before a more challenging activity is introduced. If a child requires extensive training at a certain level, therapists are encouraged to create additional variations of the particular exercise or exercises. Exercises gradually become more difficult. Parents or teachers should be advised not to jump ahead to more difficult activities without consulting the therapist.

Children with spastic cerebral palsy should practice first with ankle-foot orthotics (AFOs) and later without orthotics.

DYNAMIC STANDING BALANCE—TRANSITIONS TO STANDING, WALKING, AND STEPPING

These exercises are for children who are able to stand independently for 30 seconds but are not yet independent with transitions to and from standing nor are they walking without support. Previously, static standing balance was trained. Now movements are introduced. Sit to stand, stand to sit, stoop to stand, squat to stand, stand to squat, and stepping forward are movement sequences that require muscle coordination and timing in addition to balance. Depending on muscle tone, reflex activity, joint flexibility, perception, previous experience, and temperament of the child, some activities may be harder for one child than for another. Consequently, therapists must decide which activities are to be practiced first and which later. Parallel practice of several skills is recommended.

AFOs ensure good ground contact and ankle-foot alignment during practice. However, stiff AFOs interfere with the training of most transitional movements and should not be worn during dynamic balance training.

ADVANCED STANDING BALANCE TRAINING

These exercises are for children who are independently standing up and walking but lack the ability to stay upright when their balance is challenged or disturbed. They frequently fall, cannot balance on one foot, and may show gait abnormalities that compensate for unilateral or bilateral standing balance deficits. These activities train standing with narrow base of support, half-standing, one leg standing, and balancing on unstable surfaces. They are presented in order of difficulty with beginning skills being building blocks for later ones.

Positioning for Standing Balance Training

The most stable standing posture is one with a wide base of support and the body aligned over the center of this base of support. A wide base is created by placing the feet shoulder-width apart, slightly turned out, and flat on the floor. The body should be stacked over this base with shoulders, hips, knees, and ankles aligned over the arches of the feet. Children with cerebral palsy may need to wear AFOs in order to assume this optimal standing posture. If a child wearing AFOs stands with stiffly extended legs, forward leaning trunk, or abnormal asymmetrical posture, prerequisites for standing balance training are not met. The center of gravity is at the edge instead of over the center of the base of support. Trunk muscle activity is required to maintain standing posture, and the child is unable to relax and fine-tune balance responses.

If a child cannot assume the optimal standing posture for balance training, crouch standing is recommended. The child stands with hips, knees, and ankles flexed. The center of gravity is lowered, and the child is able to keep his or her trunk aligned over the center of the base of support. Prerequisites for balance training are met. After the child masters basic balance skills in crouch standing, straight standing balance may be practiced.

Crouch standing may be practiced barefoot, with hinged AFOs or dynamic ankle-foot orthosis (DAFOs). The child cannot crouch in stiff AFOs.

Standing With Arm Support at Furniture

PURPOSE: These activities train beginning standing balance and transitions into and out of standing. Training increases in difficulty. First, the children support themselves with their trunk and elbows. Later, the children stand with one-hand support.

Most children like to stand. Even children without balance skills want to be placed in standing positions, and they enjoy standing with parent support. The challenge is to reduce support, have the children pull to stand, and to stand independently in a safe environment.

PRACTICE SETUP: Practice on an Airex mat or soft carpeted floor. Assist or guard the child from the right or left side. Do not give back support. If you allow the child to lean against you, he will fall as soon as support is withdrawn. Instead, encourage the child to lean forward using arms for support.

1. Pull to stand and standing at a table

Encourage the child to kneel and pull to stand via half-kneel. Assist from the side and give only as much support as needed to come up. Withdraw support as soon as possible. First allow and later discourage the child from leaning with his trunk against the table. During initial standing, guard the child from the side as needed. As the child gets tired, help him drop to his knees or ease into sitting.

GOAL: The child stands at a table and moves into and out of standing with minimal assistance.

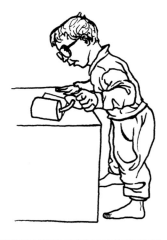

2. Pull from sit to stand and stand holding onto a stable bar

Have the child sit on a stool and hold on to the rung of a ladderbox. Encourage the child to lean forward and stand up. Briefly assist if needed. Tell her to hold on to the bar firmly and stand unassisted. Sing a song with her as encouragement to stand up longer. As the child tires, help her sit down with control.

GOAL: Holding onto a bar, the child stands up independently from a sitting position, stands for 1–3 minutes, and sits back down with control.

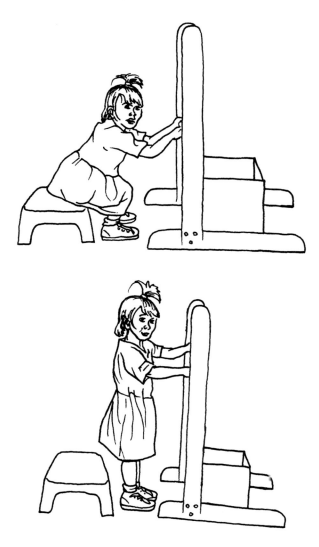

3. Standing at a table with variable arm support

Have the child pull to stand and stand at a table. Play with and encourage the child to reach with his right or left hand. Present a toy at chest level to encourage upright trunk posture.

GOAL: The child plays at a table, intermittently holding with only one hand.

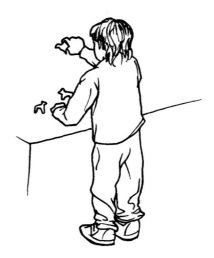

4. Standing at a table with one-arm support and trunk rotation

Have the child pull to stand and stand at a table. Play with and encourage the child to turn his trunk and reach to the side while supporting himself with one hand on the table. Practice turning to either side.

GOAL: The child independently stands while supporting himself with one arm and rotating his trunk.

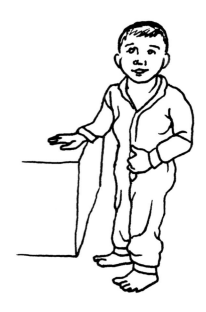

5. Stand, bend down, and return to standing

Have the child pull to stand and stand at a table. Play with and encourage the child to pick up a toy off the floor and put it on the table. If the child is reluctant, place a toy on a stool or box and have the child practice bending down a little. Use a lower box as he gains confidence. Place a toy on the floor when the child is ready for the challenge. Use a variety of toys to keep the child's interest.

GOAL: The child bends down and returns to standing, one hand supported on table, without a loss of balance.

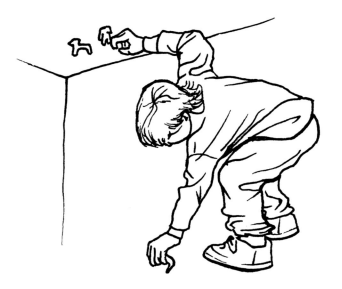

Standing With Arm Support at a Wall

PURPOSE: These activities train standing balance with reduced arm support. When standing at a piece of furniture, the child may lean forward and bear weight with her arms. At a wall, her body is aligned over her feet and all weight is carried over her legs. Her arms are used to steady her trunk and assist balancing.

PRACTICE SETUP: Practice with the child facing a wall, mirror, glass door, or other flat surface. The floor should be carpeted or covered with an Airex mat. Assist or guard the child from the side. Do not give back support.

1. Standing with both arms bracing at a wall

Ask the child to stand up at a wall via half-kneel; assist if needed. Withdraw your support and encourage her to stand independently at the wall. Assist if the child loses her balance or becomes tired.

GOAL: The child is able to stand at a wall for 30 seconds or longer.

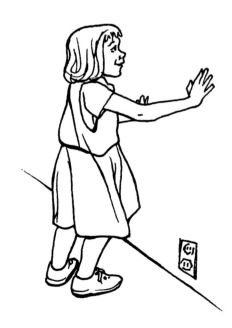

2. Standing at a wall with variable arm support and movement

Challenge the child to reduce arm support by briefly taking one hand off the wall, sliding her hands around, tapping with her hands, or moving them up or down. An enjoyable activity that incorporates these movements is playing with shaving cream on a mirror or glass door. Children like to make fingerprints with the cream, draw with it, stick foam pieces in it, or just spread it around. Cleaning up the big mess is equally fun and good exercise. Guard the child as needed.

GOAL: The child moves hands along a wall, reaches up, and bends down without a loss of balance.

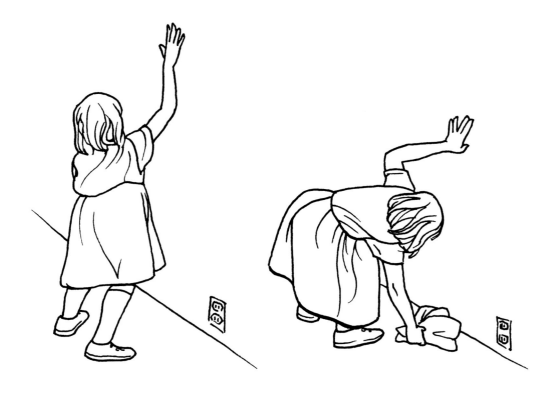

Standing With Arm Support Using Special Equipment

PURPOSE: These activities train standing balance with arm support. Special equipment is used to make activities easier, safer, or more challenging.

PRACTICE SETUP: Use appropriate equipment. Assist or guard the child from the side. Do not provide back support.

1. Standing at a ladderbox or ladder

The child pulls to stand from sitting or squatting and stands, holding onto the ladder. Provide assistance when needed. As the child gains confidence in standing independently, create play situations that challenge the child to:

a) Move her hands up or down a rung;
b) Reach with one arm up, down, out to the side, or forward; and
c) Bend down and return to standing.

GOAL: The child independently stands, holding onto a ladder with two- or one-hand support.

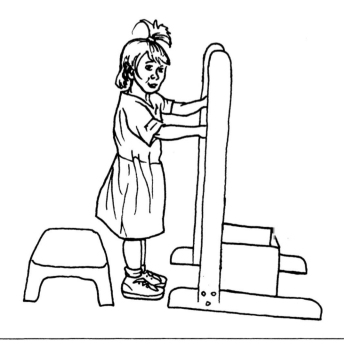

2. Standing sideways between parallel bars

For most children, it is easiest to hold onto one bar with both hands. Once the child has gained confidence in standing independently, challenge her to:

a) Take one hand off the bar and stand with one-hand support;
b) Briefly take both hands off the bar and momentarily stand without support; and
c) Stand with knees bent.

GOAL: The child independently stands sideways between parallel bars with one or both hands holding a bar. The child practices standing with her knees flexed.

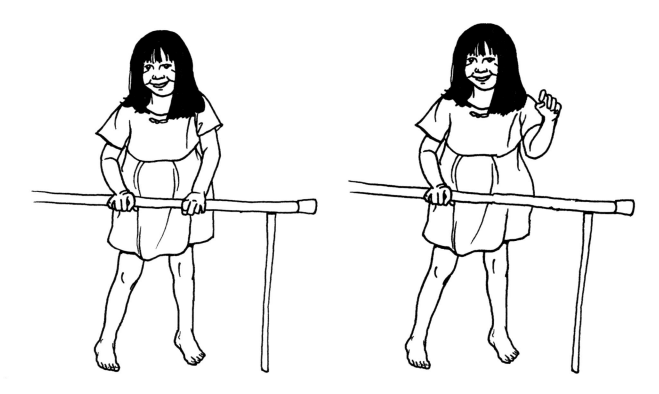

3. Standing forward between parallel bars

The child stands between the parallel bars with each hand holding onto a bar. As the child gains confidence in standing independently, challenge him to:

a) Put his open hands or only fingertips on a bar; and
b) Put his right foot forward and then try the same with his left foot.

GOAL: The child stands independently between the parallel bars. The child works on reducing arm support and changing foot position.

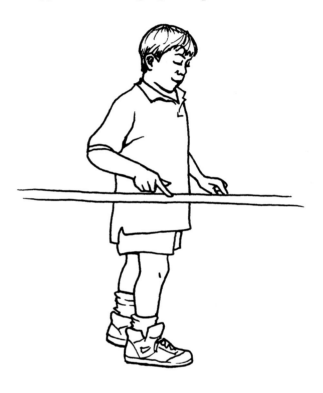

4. Standing between parallel poles

The child stands between parallel poles, holding onto a pole with each hand. Once the child has gained confidence in standing independently, challenge her to practice as in the previous activity. Various foot placements, as well as half-standing, may be practiced in parallel poles.

GOAL: The child stands independently between parallel poles. The child practices standing with reduced arm support and various foot placements.

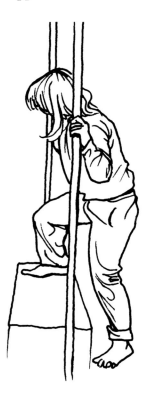

5. Standing with poles

Another way to challenge a child is to ask him to stand with unstable poles. The child may straddle a roll during practice. The roll will control wide-based foot placement and cushion an accidental fall.

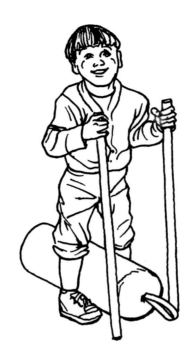

Standing With Support to Legs

PURPOSE: The child learns to balance while standing without arm support. To be successful, the child's center of mass needs to be aligned over his feet. Postural alignment is the prerequisite of independent standing. During the following activities, the child learns to achieve and maintain postural alignment. The child experiences being in alignment and losing alignment. The child learns to anticipate a loss of balance and counteract with subtle muscle activity.

PRACTICE SETUP: Practice on an Airex mat or carpeted floor. Before balance practice, help the child achieve the best possible standing posture. Shoulders and hips should be aligned over feet. For an optimal base of support, feet should be flat, slightly externally rotated, and shoulder-width apart. The child's trunk should not be touched during balance practice as this would interfere with the learning process.

1. Standing with support to legs

Assist the child with independent standing by firmly holding one or both legs at or just above the knee. Steady the child's legs and give downward pressure. This technique provides optimal floor contact with feet, reduces body sway, and challenges the child to control his trunk and hips independently in an upright position. Allow the child to play while standing for increasingly longer time periods. This activity is best done with a helper who will play with the child and spot any falls.

GOAL: The child stands and plays for several minutes with firm support to both legs or either leg.

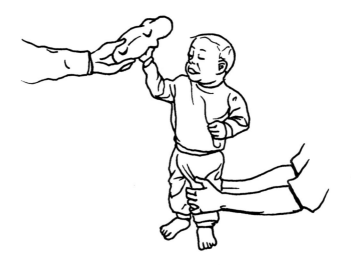

2. Standing with fading leg support

Start the activity as described in preceding one. After the child has played confidently for 1 minute, gradually release your pressure on the leg until you only lightly touch it. Allow the child to control standing posture independently. If body sway increases, resume your support. Continue play while the child is standing with intermittent support to right or left leg.

GOAL: The child stands and plays with intermittent leg support for several minutes.

3. Standing with knee support

Ask the child to raise to standing from a quadruped position, assisted by a helper if needed. Kneel behind the child. Cross your arms and firmly brace the child's right knee medially with your left hand and left knee medially with your right hand. This medial support prevents the buckling of the knees, as may happen after selective dorsal rhizotomy. Encourage the child to play while standing. Reduce your support as the child gains control.

GOAL: The child plays while standing with intermittent medial knee support.

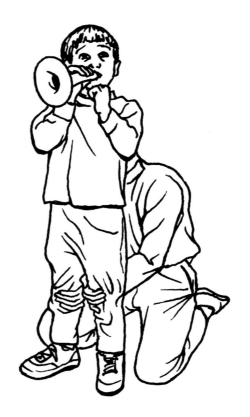

4. Standing with forefeet support

Sit on the edge of a chair and let the child stand between your legs, facing you. Place your stockinged feet over the child's forefeet. Engage the child in a play activity that keeps his hands occupied and prevents him from holding on to you. For instance, encourage the child to hold a shape drum and push shapes through the openings. Apply pressure over the child's forefeet with soles of your feet. This will provide optimal floor contact, secure the best leg position, and increase the child's stability.

GOAL: The child stands independently for several minutes with support to forefeet.

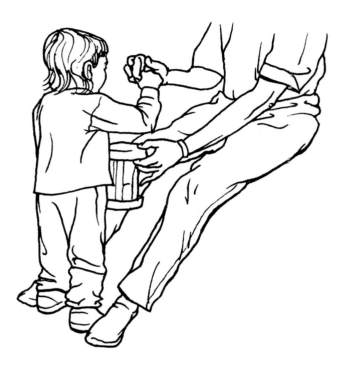

5. Standing with forefeet support and arm or body movements

Do Activity 4. During play, challenge the child to reach up and down, and encourage slight knee bends or slight bending with the trunk.

GOAL: The child stands independently with support to forefeet and moves his arms, trunk, and knees without a loss of balance.

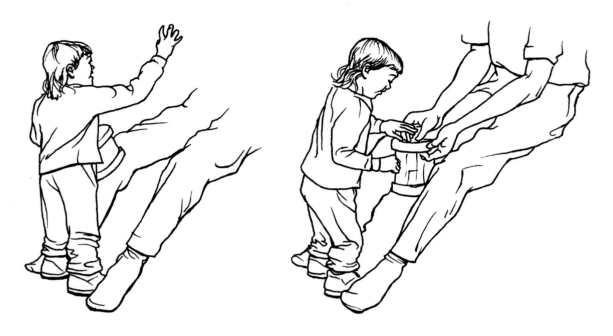

Beginning Standing Without Any Support

PURPOSE: Standing balance is trained in a safe environment. Children learn to control the position of their legs. When fearful of falling, children with cerebral palsy try to stabilize themselves by pressing their knees together. This is not helpful because, when their knees are pushed together, their legs are turned in and their heels are raised off the floor. Therefore, instead of helping children to stand, pressing their knees together reduces their base of support and triggers falling. During safe practice, children will experience this reaction. As children understand the negative consequences of pressing their knees together, they will be active participants in efforts to suppress this action and learn helpful balance reactions.

For the person working with the child, it is important to remember that the abnormal reaction is triggered by fear of falling. Therefore, it is important that practice occurs in a pleasant and safe environment, and that balance exercises are mildly challenging but not threatening to the child.

PRACTICE SETUP: Practice on an Airex mat or carpeted floor. Ask the child to stand with his feet flat, slightly externally rotated, and shoulder-width apart. Guard the child from the side or front. If the child becomes unsteady, verbally help him regain balance and optimal posture. Protect the child from falling.

1. Standing with play

Sit on the edge of a chair and let the child stand between your legs, facing you. Encourage the child to play with both hands and to not lean against you or hold on to you. Observe the child's legs. Remind him not to press his knees together. If the child loses optimal foot position, wait for him to regain balance and place his feet correctly. Assist if needed and protect the child from falls.

GOAL: The child stands independently and plays, with optimal leg position, for 1 minute or longer.

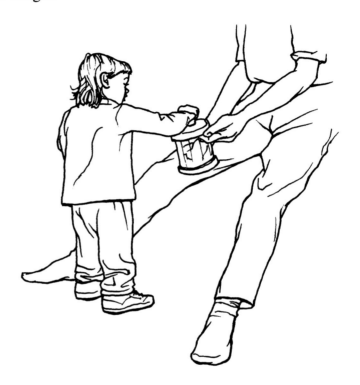

2. Standing with reach or bend down

Do the preceding activity. Play with the child and encourage him to reach up or bend down. Observe his legs. Remind the child not to press his knees together. If the child loses optimal foot position, wait for him to regain his balance and place his feet correctly.

GOAL: The child stands with optimal leg position while reaching or bending down.

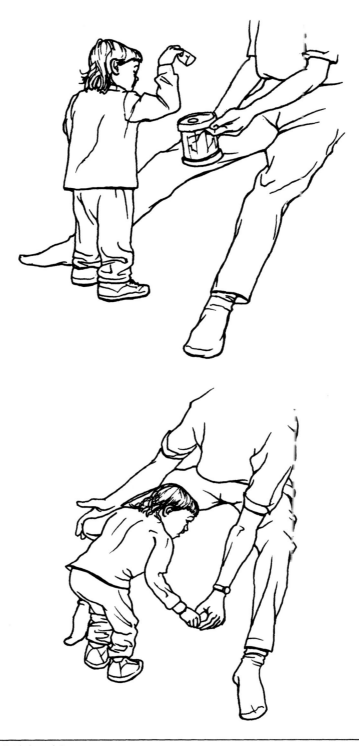

3. Standing in front of a wall

Ask the child to stand straight with his back against a wall. Once the child is comfortable standing, help him move a few inches away from the wall. Remove your support and allow the child to lean back with his buttocks against the wall. Next, challenge the child to move his hips forward and stand straight without any support. Encourage the child to count how long he stands free. If the child becomes unsteady, encourage him to move back against the wall.

GOAL: The child stands independently for 1 minute or longer.

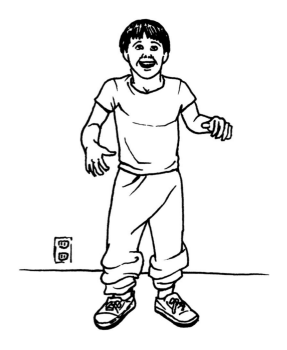

4. Standing in front of a bench

Place a bench in the middle of the room. Ask the child to crawl to it, place his hands on it, push his lower trunk up in the air, and place his feet on the floor. Assist as needed and monitor for optimal foot placement. Next, ask the child to rise to standing. Encourage the child to blow bubbles while standing for as long as possible. If the child becomes unsteady or tired, encourage him to lower his trunk and catch himself with his arms on the bench.

GOAL: Using a bench, the child rises independently to standing, stands, and lowers himself with control.

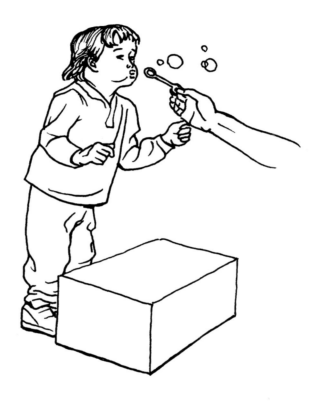

Beginning Standing Without Protection From a Fall

PURPOSE: The child learns to maintain standing balance during a variety of activities. Training occurs without protection from a fall. The child is challenged to become aware of unsteadiness and counteract and prevent falls to the best of his or her ability.

PRECAUTION: These activities should be practiced only with children who control falls well enough not to get hurt when falling.

PRACTICE SETUP: Practice on an Airex mat or carpeted floor. Ask the child to stand with her feet flat, slightly externally rotated, and shoulder-width apart. If the child becomes unsteady, wait for her to regain balance and optimal posture. Provide verbal prompts if needed.

1. Standing with play

Help the child stand up in the middle of the room and assume optimal standing posture. After the child stands independently, encourage the child to engage in a play activity that requires minimal arm or trunk movement. Looking at colorful beads in a baby toy or singing into a make-believe microphone may be fun.

GOAL: The child stands independently for several minutes without becoming unsteady.

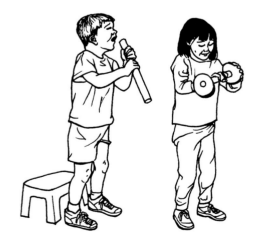

2. Standing with reach

Help the child stand up in the middle of the room and assume optimal standing posture. Engage the child in a play activity and encourage him to reach up with his right or left hand. As the child's confidence improves, ask him to raise both arms.

GOAL: The child maintains standing balance while lifting one or both arms.

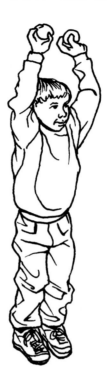

3. Standing, bending down, and return to standing

Ask the child to stand up in the middle of the room. Assist if needed. Once the child has assumed optimal standing posture, place a toy on the floor within easy reach. Encourage the child to pick up the toy. Use a large, easy-to-grasp toy first. As the child improves, challenge her to bend down farther and pick up small things.

GOAL: The child maintains balance while bending down and returning to standing.

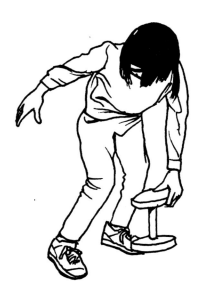

4. Playing ball

Playing ball is fun and motivating. Gentle ball play can be used for initial balance training. Ask the child to stand with optimal standing posture and use a lightweight, medium-size ball. First, hand the ball to the child and tell him to throw it back to you. Next, roll the ball and encourage the child to pick it up. At a later play session, you may try to throw the ball and ask the child to catch it.

GOAL: The child maintains balance while reaching for, throwing, or catching a ball.

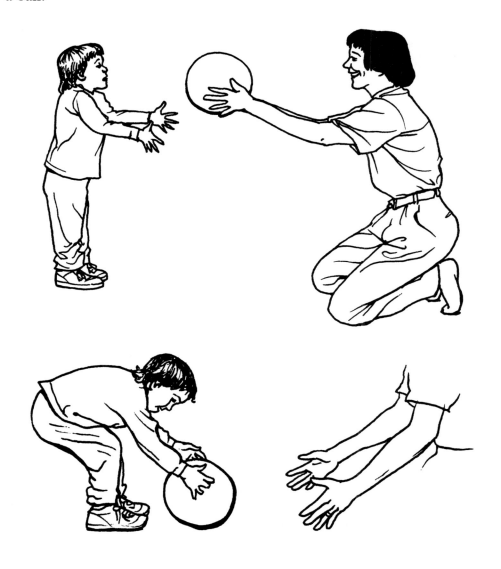

5. Punching and pushing

Punching and pushing a large, heavy object is fun and requires counteraction. It is good beginning balance training. Tumble Form rolls or a rolled and tied-up carpet piece both work well with this activity.

GOAL: The child maintains balance when punching or pushing a heavy roll.

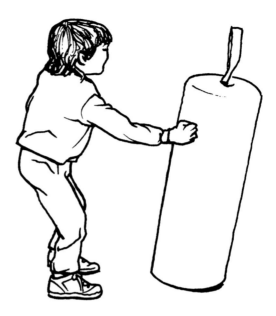

Crouch Standing

PURPOSE: The child learns to stand barefoot with his feet flat and to balance in standing. These activities are for children with cerebral palsy who toe stand or stand with their trunk leaning forward, have stiffly extended legs, and have minimal or no standing balance. Asked to stand straight with feet flat, the child loses balance and falls backward. When taught to stand with knees and hips flexed, the child gains the ability to align his shoulders and hips over flat feet. Now, with the center of mass aligned over the base of support, balance training is possible. After the child has gained balance in crouch standing, straight standing can be practiced.

PRACTICE SETUP: Practice on an Airex mat or carpeted floor. Begin by having the child play in squat position with assistance. Give the child time to relax into full plantar flexion with his feet flat. Next, help the child stand up and balance. Secure a Tumble Forms roll in front of the child's shins and have him stand crouched with his lower legs leaning against and supported by the roll. His feet should be flat, shoulder-width apart, and slightly turned out.

1. Crouch standing with shin and arm support

Be in front of the child and hold up an interesting toy. Encourage the child to hold onto the toy and play quietly as long as possible.

GOAL: The child plays in crouch standing with arm support for 1 minute or longer.

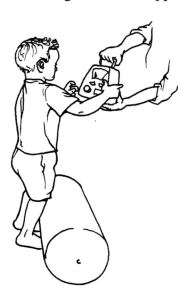

2. Free crouch standing with shin support

The child crouch stands with his shins stabilized against a Tumble Forms roll. Sit across from the child and encourage him to play with both hands, balancing without arm support. Allow the child to play quietly as long as possible.

GOAL: The child plays in crouch standing without any support for 1 minute or longer.

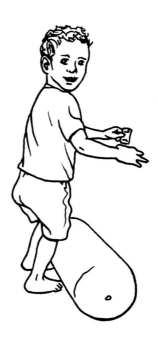

3. Independent crouch standing without support

Do the preceding activity. Once the child stands comfortably, gently move the roll away from his shins and encourage him to stand and play without support. Observe the child's legs; remind him not to press his knees together. If the child loses optimal foot position, wait for him to relax and regain optimal posture; assist as needed. Encourage the child to stand as long as possible.

GOAL: The child crouch stands independently for 1 minute or longer.

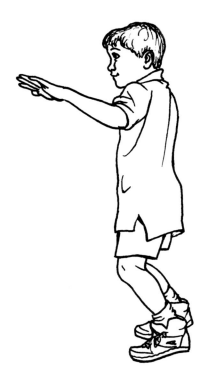

PRECAUTION: It is important that the child does not fall during the exercises. In order to improve, the child must gain confidence. Progress slowly. Any unexpected and uncontrolled fall, even if the child is not hurt, may cause a setback.

Play in Squatting

PURPOSE: This activity trains balance with feet flat and a low center of gravity.

PRACTICE SETUP: Practice in the middle of the room away from furniture.

ACTIVITY: Place the child's favorite toy on the floor. Assist the child as needed to squat down and play. Give balance support until the child relaxes, has his feet flat and slightly turned out, and the center of his body is over his feet. Slowly withdraw your support and encourage the child to play in a squat for 1 minute or longer.

GOAL: The child plays independently while squatting.

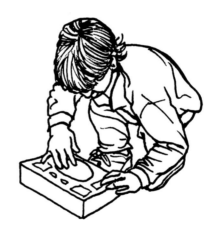

Balance Training With Crutches

PURPOSE: The first two activities train the child to stay upright with crutches. The last three activities challenge the crutch-walking child. They improve balance and coordination as he or she maneuvers with crutches.

PRACTICE SETUP: Practice on an Airex mat or carpet. Give standby assistance. Have the child wear a gait belt or safety helmet if necessary.

1. Standing with crutches

Help the child stand with good alignment, leaning on crutches. Slowly withdraw your support and challenge the child to balance for 10 counts while you guard closely. Support and praise the child after the task is accomplished. Repeat the exercise several times.

NOTE: Initial standing with crutches requires concentration and produces anxiety. Pauses with physical support and praise are important to relax tight muscles and build confidence.

GOAL: The child stands with ease, leaning on crutches, for 10 seconds.

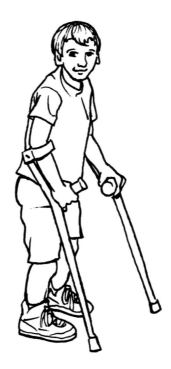

2. Crutch standing with weight shift

Have the child stand unassisted with crutches. Place a balloon in front of the left crutch. Tell the child to lean on the right crutch and toss the balloon with the left crutch; do several repetitions. Closely watch the child at all times and give balance assistance as needed. Next, place the balloon on the other side and have the child toss the balloon with the right crutch.

GOAL: The child successfully shifts weight and lifts either crutch.

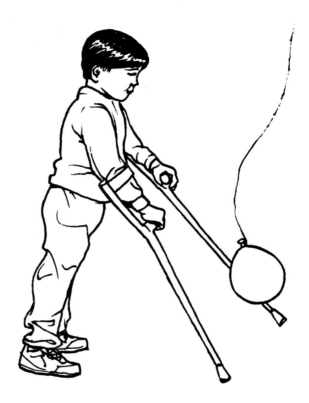

3. Turning with crutches

Place a large hoop on the floor and ask the child to step inside it with his crutches. Challenge the child to turn around without placing his feet or crutches outside the hoop. After the child successfully accomplishes the task, repeat the activity with a smaller hoop.

GOAL: The child is able to negotiate tight corners with crutches.

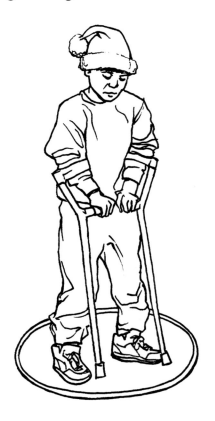

4. Stepping over a barrier with crutches

Place a stick horizontally in front of the child's crutches and challenge him to step over it. Tell the child to move his crutches first, and then his feet, over the stick. After the task is accomplished, increase the difficulty of the exercise by having the child step over boards of different widths and heights.

GOAL: The child is able to negotiate barriers with crutches.

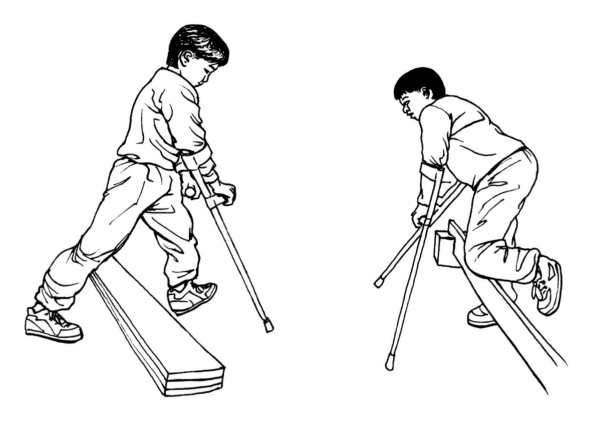

5. Half-standing with crutches

Place a platform 4″ high in front of the child and ask him to put one foot on the platform; assist as needed. Challenge the child to balance independently for 10 counts. Repeat five times. Then practice with the other foot on the platform.

GOAL: The child is able to balance with most of his weight over one foot and arm support on crutches.

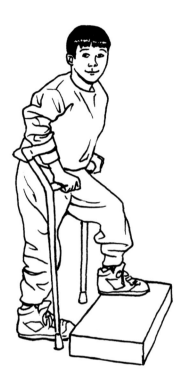

6. Practice functional skills with crutches

Have the child crutch-walk up and down an incline, on grass, up and down
a curb, and up and down stairs.

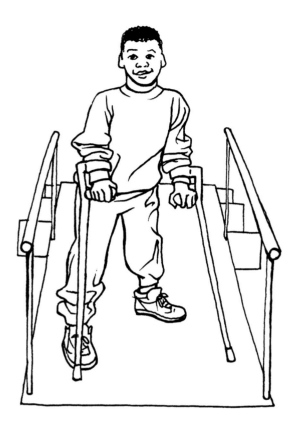

Dynamic Standing Balance— Transitions to Standing, Walking, and Stepping

Balance During Transition to and From Standing

Sit to Stand

PURPOSE: The child learns to shift weight forward and move from sit to stand without arm support. The child learns to sit down with control.

PRACTICE SETUP: Have the child sit on a stool in the middle of the room, away from furniture. Stand in front of the child. Tell or help the child to place his legs in optimal position: knees apart and aligned with hips, and feet flat and slightly turned out. Have seats of different heights available. Because it is easier to stand up from a high bench than a low one, use a higher bench for initial practice and increasingly lower ones later. If different-sized benches are unavailable, a sturdy box or several large books stacked up and tied together may be good substitutes.

1. Standing up and sitting down, holding onto a hoop

Encourage the child to hold onto a hoop, lean his trunk forward, and stand up. Monitor the child's legs. Remind the child not to press his knees together while coming up. Have the child practice sitting down slowly and softly. Do numerous repetitions. As he improves, relax your hold on the hoop and challenge the child to move up or down with minimal support.

GOAL: The child stands up and sits down with minimal arm support.

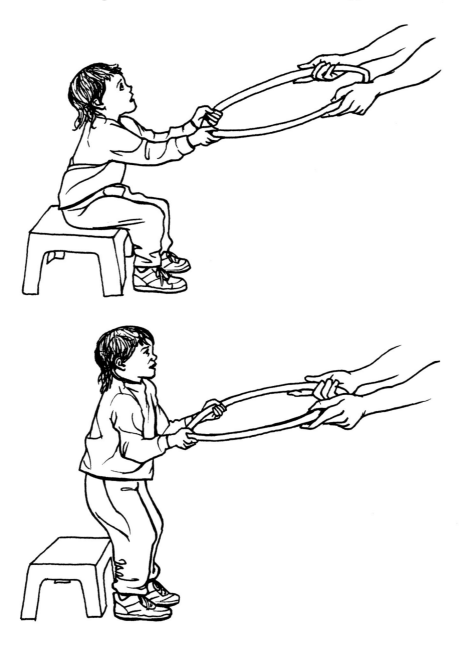

2. Standing up and sitting down with one-hand support

Place several play tokens on the floor. Encourage the child to pick up a token, lean forward, stand up while pushing off with one hand, and place the token into a slot. Monitor the child's legs and remind him not to press his knees together while coming up. Later, tell the child to sit down slowly and softly to get another token. Practice first from a high bench and then from low ones. Encourage the child to push off with either hand.

GOAL: The child stands up and sits down with the support of his right or left arm.

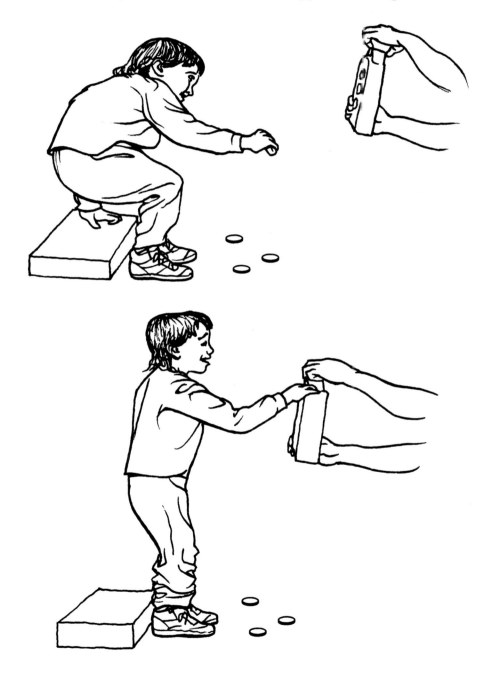

3. Learning to stand up without arm support

Ask the child to hug a favorite stuffed toy firmly, lean forward, and stand up with the animal. Guard or briefly assist as needed. Monitor the child's legs and remind him not to press his knees together while coming up. Later, tell the child to sit down slowly and softly. Practice for numerous repetitions using another stuffed toy, doll, or ball for variety. Withdraw all support as the child improves.

GOAL: The child stands up and sits down independently without arm support.

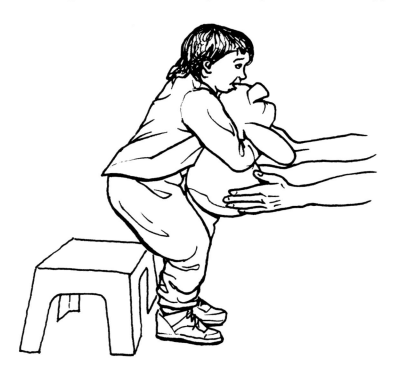

4. Standing up and sitting down without arm support

Choose a play activity the child likes and have the child stand up or sit down at each turn. Monitor the child's legs. If needed, remind the child to keep his knees apart. If the child loses optimal foot placement, wait for him to "fix" his feet. Do numerous repetitions, encouraging smooth, graded movements.

GOAL: The child stands up and sits down with control and no arm support.

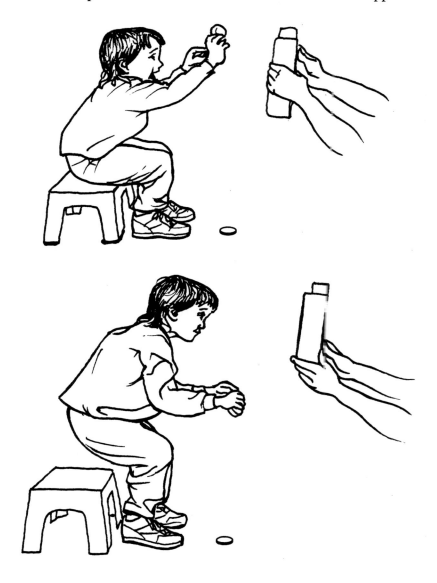

Quadruped to Stand

PURPOSE: The child learns to stand up in the middle of the room without any support. This is a significant functional milestone.

PRACTICE SETUP: Practice in the middle of the room, away from furniture. The floor should be carpeted or covered with an Airex mat. Be at the side or in front of the child.

1. Pushing to stand from a bench

Place a bench in the middle of the room. Ask the child to place his hands on the bench, push his lower trunk up in the air, and place his feet on the floor. Assist as needed and monitor for optimal foot placement: feet flat, slightly turned out, and shoulder-width apart. Encourage the child to rise to standing. First practice with a high bench and then increasingly lower ones.

GOAL: The child stands up independently by pushing off a low bench.

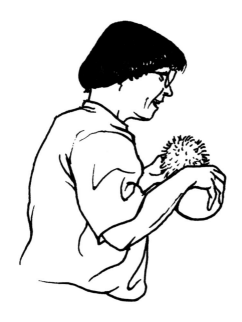
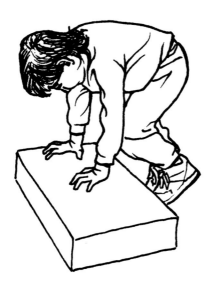

2. Pushing to stand from the floor

Encourage the child to raise his lower trunk and place his feet on the floor from the four-point position. Remind him to place his feet shoulder-width apart. It may not be possible and is not necessary that feet are flat in this position. Encourage the child to rise to standing. During initial practice, it may help the child to place one or both hands on a book or toy. As the child improves, provide opportunities for independent practice. No longer monitor foot placement. Allow the child to experiment with coming up from various positions.

GOAL: The child stands up independently in the middle of the room.

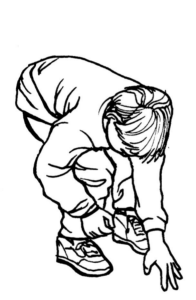 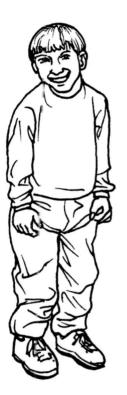

Squat to Stand and Stand to Squat

PURPOSE: The child learns to stand up from squatting and to lower himself to a squat. This activity trains lower extremity coordination and balance.

PRACTICE SETUP: Practice in the middle of the room, away from furniture. The floor should be carpeted or covered with an Airex mat.

1. Stand to squat with arm support

Have the child stand with his feet flat, slightly turned out, and shoulder-width apart. Stand across from the child and encourage him to play with the toy you hold. Slowly lower the toy and entice the child to bend his knees, crouch, and finally to squat and play. If needed, remind or assist the child to keep his knees apart and feet in optimal position. Do numerous repetitions.

GOAL: The child slowly moves from stand to squat with minimal arm support.

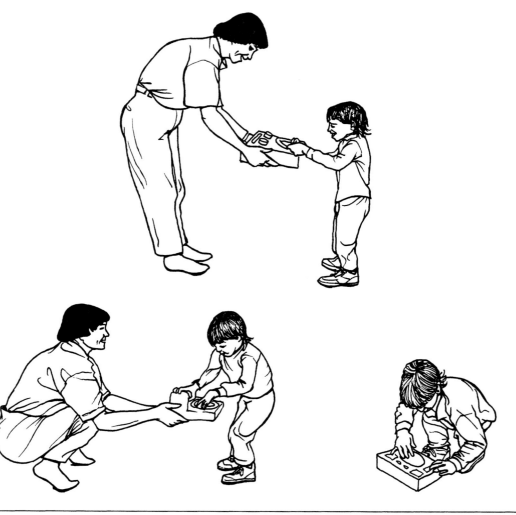

2. Squat to stand with arm support

Have the child play in squat with his knees apart, feet flat, and slightly turned out. Slowly raise the toy and encourage the child to stand up. Monitor the child's feet. Remind or assist the child to keep them in optimal position. Do numerous repetitions.

GOAL: The child stands up with minimal arm support.

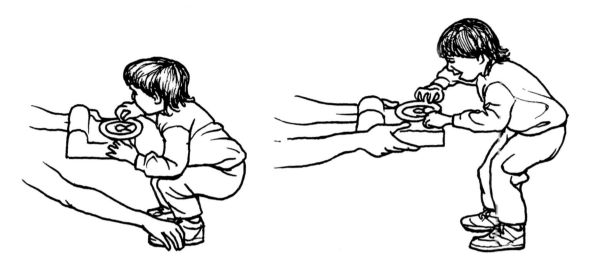

3. Practice without arm support

Create a play situation that requires moving from stand to squat and from squat to stand. Reaching for marbles, blocks, or toy animals and setting them up on the floor may be fun. Monitor the child's legs. Encourage the child to keep his feet flat, slightly turned out, and apart. Spot the child as needed. As the child improves, provide opportunity for independent play.

GOAL: The child moves independently from squat to stand and vice versa.

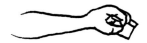

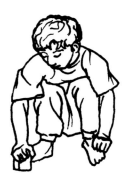

Beginning Walking

Walking With Arm Support

PURPOSE: The child learns to step forward while holding on with arms. The activities are presented in order of decreasing support.

PRACTICE SETUP: Practice in an open, carpeted space.

1. Pushing a toy cart

Let the child hold onto a toy cart and walk with it. If the cart rolls too fast and makes the child trip and fall, weigh the cart down with sandbags. Practicing on thick carpet or while going up a slight incline may be other options. Encourage the child to keep his feet apart in order not to trip.

GOAL: The child stays upright and steps while leaning on a mobile support.

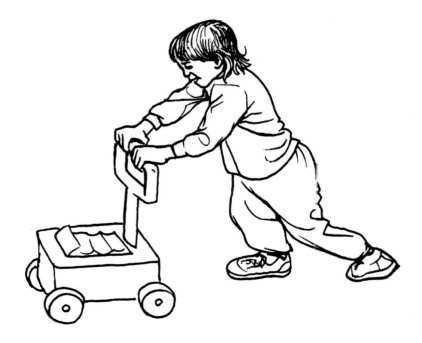

2. Walking with sticks

Have the child stand with his feet flat, slightly turned out, and shoulder-width apart. Stand in front of the child and present two sticks. Encourage the child to hold onto the sticks and step with you. Remind the child not to turn his feet in, as it makes him trip. As the child improves, reduce your hold on the sticks.

GOAL: The child walks 50 feet holding onto a stick.

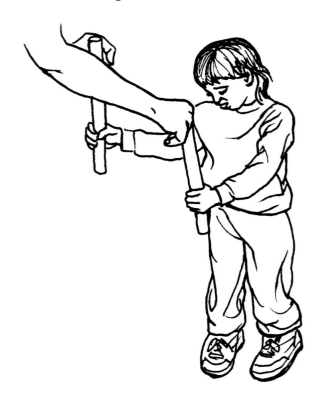

3. Walking with a hoop

Have the child stand with his feet flat, slightly turned out, and shoulder-width apart. Stand in front and present a hoop to the child. Encourage the child to hold onto the hoop and walk with you. Remind the child not to turn his feet in.

GOAL: The child walks 50 feet holding onto a hoop.

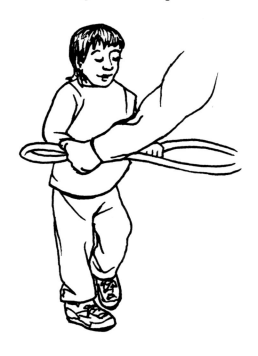

Walking With Minimal or No Arm Support

PURPOSE: The child learns to walk a short distance independently.

PRACTICE SETUP: Practice in an open space or as directed.

1. Walking with one hand against a wall

Have the child stand close to a wall with his feet flat, slightly turned out, and shoulder-width apart. Ask the child to brace himself with one hand against the wall and walk to you. Remind the child to walk slowly and to keep his feet straight. Encourage the child to walk increasingly longer distances. The child should practice with either hand against the wall.

GOAL: The child walks with his right or left hand braced against a wall for 30 feet.

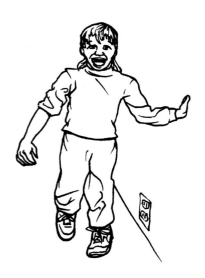

2. Stand, walk a few steps, stand

Place an attractive toy on a Tumble Forms roll or tall, narrow box. Help the child stand with good posture and balance 1–2 feet away. His feet should be flat, slightly turned out, and shoulder-width apart. Encourage the child to walk to the roll, stand still, and get the toy. Do numerous repetitions of one, two, or three independent steps. You want to build confidence and balance.

GOAL: The child starts, stops, and walks one to three steps independently.

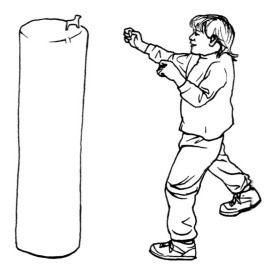

3. Stand, walk, stand

Practice as in the preceding activity. Slowly increase the distance and encourage the child to walk more steps at a time. If the child starts to lose his balance, ask him to pause, "fix" his feet, balance, and then go on.

GOAL: The child walks slowly for increasingly longer distances.

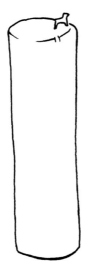
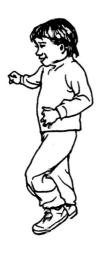

4. Walking while straddling a divider*

Help the child to straddle a divider and ask him to place his feet flat, slightly turned out, and apart. Once the child has gained balance, encourage him to walk slowly to you. The divider will require the child to keep his feet apart and step with control while discouraging adduction and internal rotation. If the child does not have the balance skills needed, practice first with slight support to his hips or let the child hold onto a hoop. (See walking with arm support.)

GOAL: The child walks a short distance with control and improved balance.

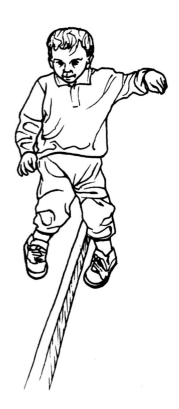

---

*Divider is commercially available or may be constructed using a 2″ x 4″ board.

Beginning Independent Walking

PURPOSE: The child's walking balance and coordination are trained. The child learns to walk in increasingly more challenging situations.

PRACTICE SETUP: Practice in an open space or as directed.

1. Walking on uneven surfaces

Practice with the child to:

a) Walk on grass; and
b) Walk on a thick exercise mat. Practice at home by placing a mattress on the floor and encouraging the child to walk on it. Help the child step on or off the mattress if needed. Guard the child from tripping off the mattress during the activity.

GOAL: The child does not fall when walking on grass or a mattress.

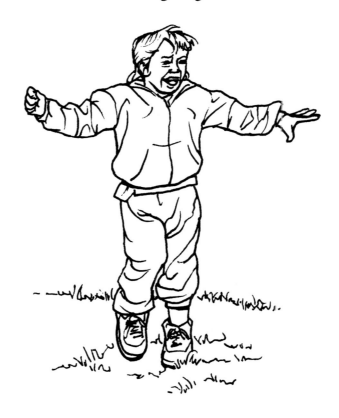

2. Walking up and down an incline

Encourage the child to walk up and down an incline, such as a wheelchair ramp. Hold the child by one hand first and later ask the child to walk independently.

GOAL: The child walks up and down an incline without falling.

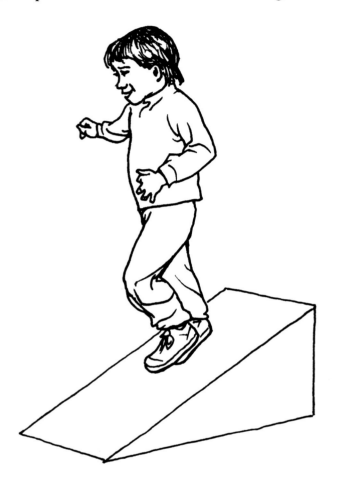

3. Walking while straddling a barrier

Place a Poly Beam, wooden slats, or thick rope on the floor. (Wooden toy train tracks may also work.) Ask the child to walk with one foot on either side of the item and not to step on it. This exercise trains the child to keep her feet apart and walk in a straight line.

GOAL: The child walks 30 feet without stepping on the barrier.

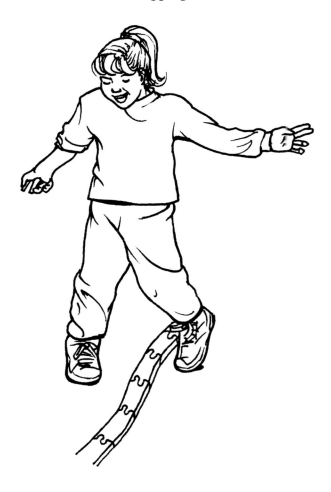

4. Walking between barriers

Make a lane 2 feet wide by putting wide ribbons, wooden slats, or a thick rope on the floor. Ask the child to walk in the lane without stepping on the side barriers. Once the child has gained confidence and does this well, make the lane narrower. This exercise trains the child to walk straight and step forward with a narrow base of support.

GOAL: The child walks with an increasingly narrower base of support.

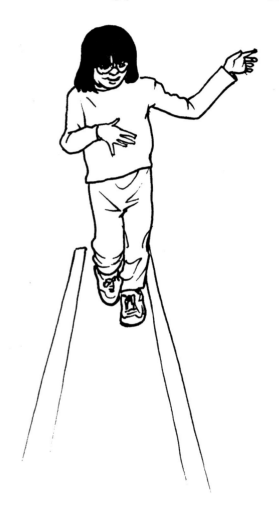

5. Stepping into a hoop and turning around

Place a large hoop on the floor and ask the child to step inside. Challenge the child to turn around without stepping on or outside the hoop. If the child is successful, do the activity with a smaller hoop. Guard the child as needed.

GOAL: The child turns around in small space independently.

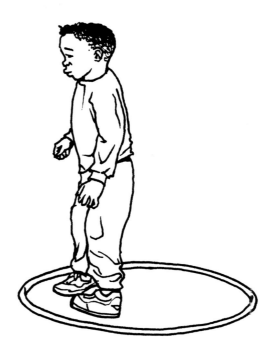

6. Stepping over a barrier

Have the child stand with his feet flat, slightly turned out, and apart. Place a thick rope in front of the child's feet and challenge him to step over it. After the task is accomplished, increase the difficulty of the exercise. Have the child step over increasingly wider or higher barriers. For instance, ask the child to step over a 2″ rod, 4″ Poly Beam, 6″ board, wooden train track, or stuffed animals set in a row. Guard the child as needed.

GOAL: The child steps over the barrier without a loss of balance.

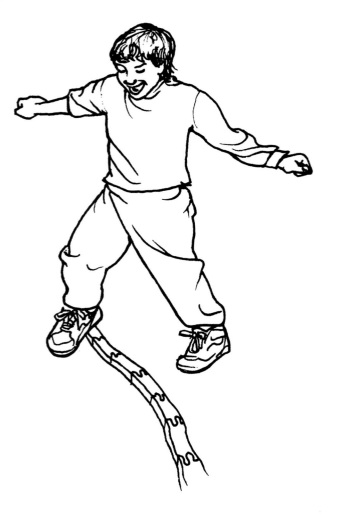

Sidestepping With Support

PURPOSE: Protective sidestepping is an automatic reaction of our lower extremities whenever our balance is seriously challenged. Stepping to the side widens our base of support and helps us regain our balance. Children with cerebral palsy show no, or delayed, sidestepping. Training of sidestepping will benefit them.

PRACTICE SETUP: During sidestepping, children need to shift most of their weight to one side and firmly stand and balance on that side in order to lift the other foot off the floor and sidestep. Sidestepping is facilitated by inducing weight shifts and by supporting the standing leg. Provide a physical prompt to move the leg if necessary.

1. Sidestepping along furniture

Practice sidestepping between parallel bars or along chest-high furniture. Assist or guard the child on the left side when stepping to the right and vice versa. Reduce your assistance as the child improves.

GOAL: The child independently sidesteps to the right and left side along furniture.

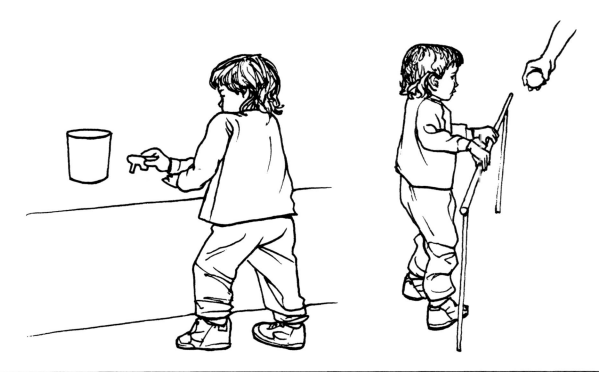

---

2. Sidestepping with arm support against a wall

Practice sidestepping along a wall. Assist or guard the child on the left side when stepping to the right and vice versa. Reduce assistance as the child improves.

GOAL: The child sidesteps independently to the right and left side along a wall.

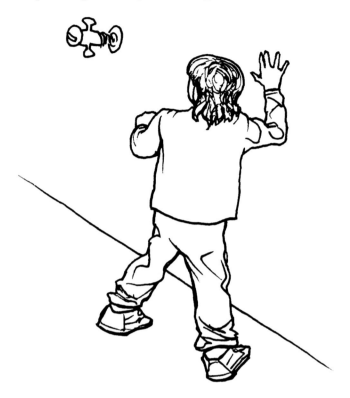

3. Sidestepping with back support

Practice sidestepping with the child's back against a wall Assist or guard the child on the left side when stepping to the right; charge sides when the child steps to the left. Reduce assistance as the child improves.

GOAL: The child sidesteps independently to the left or right side with his back against the wall.

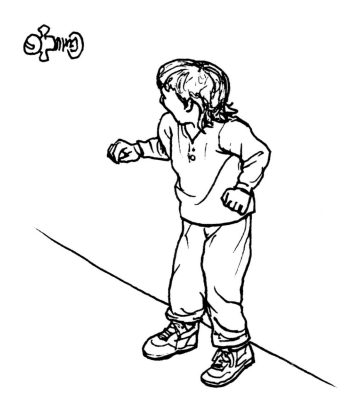

Sidestepping With Minimal Arm Support

PURPOSE: Protective sidestepping is an automatic reaction of our lower extremities whenever our balance is seriously challenged. Stepping to the side widens the base of support, helps us regain our balance, and prevents us from falling. Children with cerebral palsy show no, or delayed, sidestepping. Training of sidestepping will benefit them.

PRACTICE SETUP: The child stands in the middle of a carpeted room, away from furniture.

1. Sidestepping holding hands

Stand across from the child and hold hands. Ask the child to kick his leg out to the side and step to the side with you. Sing a song as you go to the right and then to the left side.

GOAL: The child sidesteps with arm support.

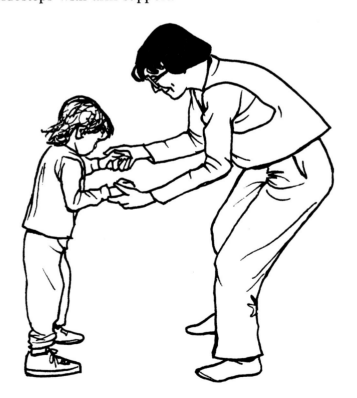

---

2. Sidestepping holding onto a large object

Stand across from the child and ask her to help you carry a Tumble Forms roll or large box. You may use several rolls or boxes to build a house or tower. Later you may play cleanup. Practice sidestepping to the left and right side.

GOAL: The child sidesteps in a functional situation.

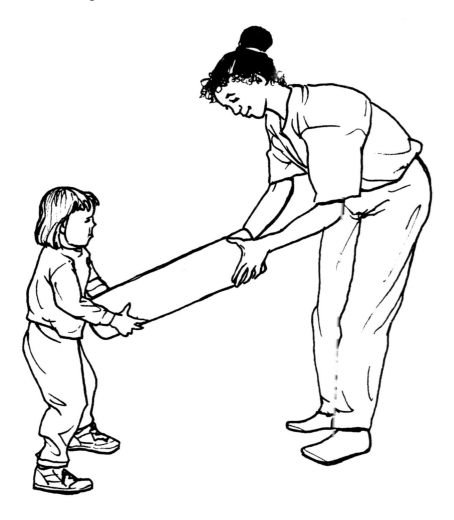

3. Sidestepping holding onto a hoop

Stand across from the child, holding a hoop. Ask the child to hold onto the hoop and sidestep with you. Sing a song while you step to the right or left side.

GOAL: The child sidesteps with minimal balance support.

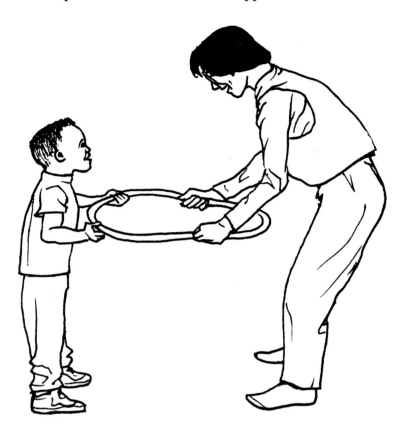

Independent Sidestepping

PURPOSE: Protective sidestepping is an automatic reaction of our lower extremities whenever our balance is seriously challenged. Stepping to the side widens the base of support, helps us regain our balance, and prevents us from falling. Children with cerebral palsy show no, or delayed, sidestepping. Training of sidestepping will benefit them.

PRACTICE SETUP: The child stands in the middle of the room, away from furniture.

1. Stepping to the side and returning to the starting position

The child stands with his feet fairly close together. Put a sticker on the floor next to the child's left foot. Encourage the child to step on it and then off. "Make the picture go away! . . . Let me see it again!" Do 10 repetitions with either foot. Use different stickers for variety.

GOAL: The child sidesteps and returns to the starting position without a loss of balance.

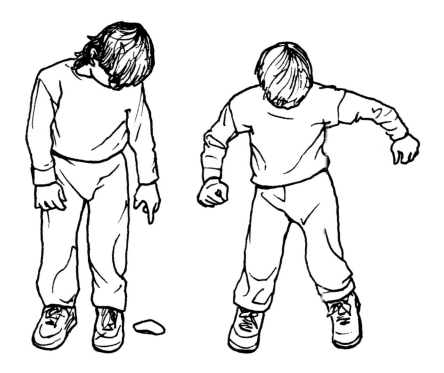

2. Continuous sidestepping

a) Create a situation that induces the child to sidestep. For instance, build a "bridge" with a board or balance beam and encourage the child to step along it and get the animals off the bridge or place them there.

b) Challenge the child to sidestep along a line.

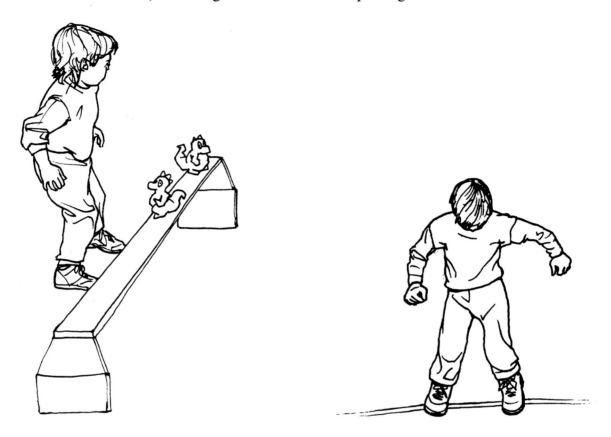

GOAL: The child sidesteps independently for 10 feet or longer to either side.

3. Spontaneous sidestepping during play

Play ball or balloon toss with the child. First toss a ball into the child's immediate range. As the child relaxes and enjoys the game, toss the ball a little to the right or left side and encourage him to step to the side to catch it.

GOAL: The child spontaneously sidesteps during play.

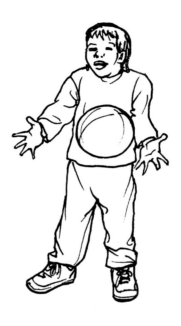

4. Protective sidestepping practice

Ask the child to stand with his feet as close together as possible. Give a brief push at the left hip and encourage the child to sidestep quickly with his right foot and not fall down. Practice toward the left side the same way. Guard the child well during this exercise. Have another person assist if needed.

GOAL: The child stays upright by quickly stepping to the side.

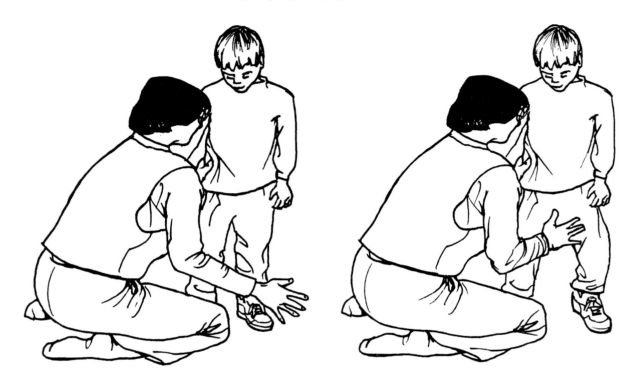

Back Stepping

PURPOSE: The child learns to step backward. Being able to step back has functional importance. It helps the child to get around in small places. Also, with backward loss of balance, a quick step back protects the child from falling.

PRACTICE SETUP: Practice in the middle of the room or as directed.

1. Back stepping with guidance

Holding hands, stand next to the child in front of a mirror. Demonstrate the movement while telling the child to lift one foot, kick it backward, and step back. Practice together, encouraging the child to look into the mirror and watch the steps.

GOAL: The child steps backward with verbal, visual, and balance assistance.

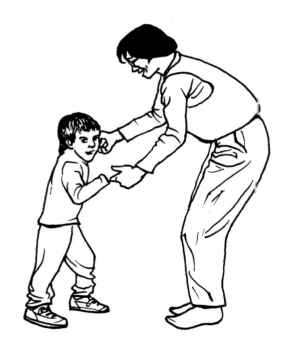

2. Back stepping with one hand against the wall

Practice in a hallway. Ask the child to back step with one hand braced against the wall. Count backward steps, encouraging the child to do 5, 10, or more steps in a row.

GOAL: The child takes 30 steps back with one hand against the wall.

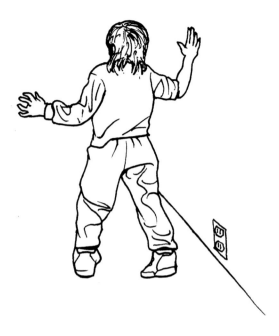

3. Back stepping holding onto a hoop

Stand or kneel across from the child, holding a hoop. Ask the child to hold onto the hoop and walk backward with you. Encourage the child to kick his leg far back with each step.

GOAL: The child walks backward, holding onto a hoop for balance support.

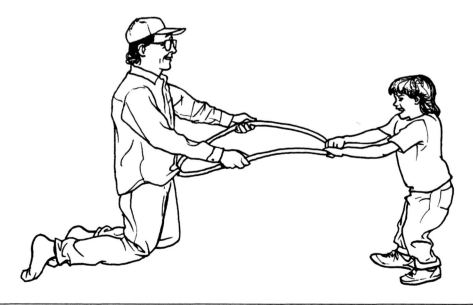

4. Independent back stepping

a) Practice back stepping as described in the preceding activity, only this time do not have the child hold onto your hands or a hoop.

b) Play falling down. Make a soft pile out of beanbag chairs, pillows, blankets, or other suitable things. Have the child stand 2 feet away with his back toward the soft pile. Tell the child to slowly walk backward and, as the child feels the pile with his foot, to have fun falling into it. If the child likes this game, have him walk increasingly longer distances backward.

GOAL: The child back steps independently for 10 feet.

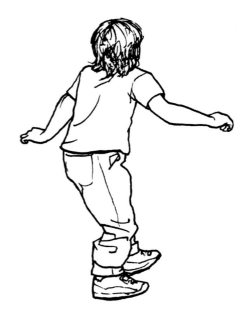

5. Training of protective back stepping with loss of balance backward

Have the child stand with his feet flat, slightly turned out, and apart. Give a gentle, brief push to the child's trunk and encourage him to step back quickly in order not to fall. Guard the child well. Have another person assisting you if needed.

GOAL: The child uses a protective back step to stay upright.

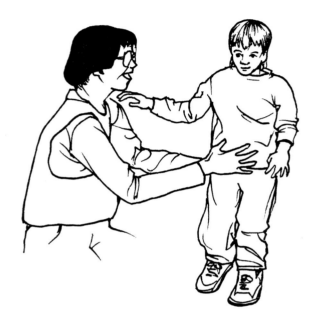

Advanced Standing Balance

Balance Practice on a Stool

PURPOSE: The child learns to balance while standing with a narrow base of support. At the same time, activities train gradual ankle and knee flexion and extension in weight bearing. The child learns to maintain her balance while her center of gravity moves up and down.

When standing on a stool, the child cannot use protective stepping to keep her balance, which makes this a challenging activity.

PRACTICE SETUP: The size of the stool depends on the child's foot size and skill level. It is easier to balance on a large platform than a small one. Yet, the platform may not be smaller than the child's feet. Neither her heels nor her toes should hang over the edge. If the child is afraid of heights, a large, sturdy book may be used. All exercises should be practiced first on a wider platform and later on a smaller one. Closely guard the child from the side or front. Improve safety by placing the stool in front of a bed or low couch.

1. Quiet standing

Help the child step onto the stool and stand with her feet flat and straight forward or slightly turned out. After the child has gained balance, slowly withdraw your support. Challenge the child to stand independently for five counts, 10 counts, and so on.

GOAL: The child balances for 30 seconds or longer.

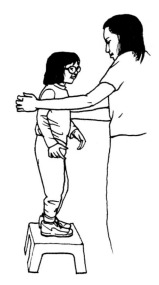

2. Standing with play

Help the child step onto the stool and stand with his feet flat and straight forward or slightly turned out. Withdraw support as the child gains balance. Encourage the child to blow different whistles, blow bubbles, or play with a toy. Once the child has gained confidence, challenge the child to reach up or out for a whistle or pop the bubbles you blow. Carefully grade activities. Watch and guard the child at all times.

GOAL: The child balances on a stool for 2 minutes while quietly playing or reaching.

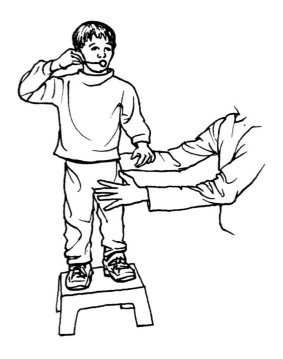

3. Stand to crouch

Have the child stand on a stool with her feet flat and straight forward or slightly turned out. Place a toy on the stool next to her feet or on the floor and challenge the child to pick it up. Closely guard the child. If she is unable to get to the toy, hold it a little higher at first. Have the child crouch down only as far as she can without raising her heels. Verbally cue the child to keep her feet flat and to move slowly up or down. Do many repetitions, using different toys for variety.

GOAL: The child lowers to a crouch and stands again without a loss of balance.

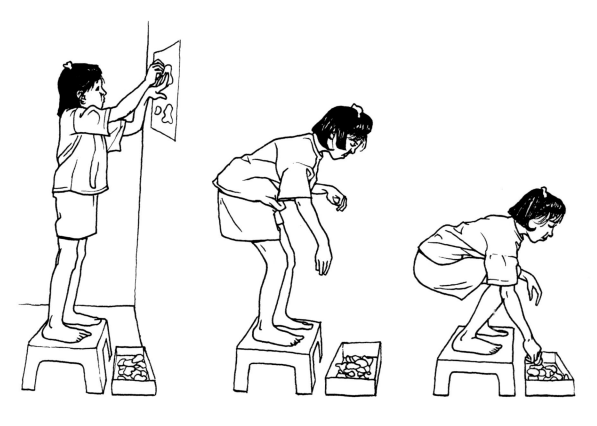

4. Stand to squat

Have the child stand on a stool with her feet flat and straight forward or slightly turned out. Place a stacking cone on the floor in front of the stool. Offer a ring to the child and encourage her to squat down and stack it on the cone. Verbally cue the child to keep her feet flat and move slowly down or up. Do numerous repetitions. This activity becomes more difficult if the stacking cone is placed to the right or left side of the stool.

GOAL: The child lowers to a squat and stands again without a loss of balance.

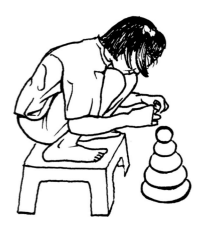

5. Stand and reach high

Have the child stand on a stool with her feet flat and straight forward or slightly turned out. Hold a toy up, slightly out of reach. Challenge the child to stretch, come up onto her forefeet, and reach for it. Carefully watch and guard the child. Do numerous repetitions. You may also alternate reaching high with crouching or squatting.

GOAL: The child rises to her forefeet without a loss of balance.

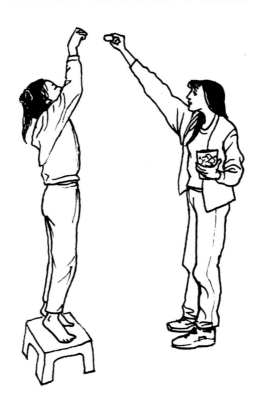

Balance With Feet in Various Positions

PURPOSE: The child learns to balance with a small base of support, with a narrow and long base of support, and with most of her weight over her heels.

PRACTICE SETUP: Practice in the middle of a carpeted room or on an Airex mat. Guard the child from the side as needed.

1. Standing with heels together

Ask the child to stand with his heels as close together as possible. His forefeet are apart because his legs should be slightly turned out. Count how long he can balance in this position. As the child gains confidence, challenge him to play basketball.

GOAL: The child stands with his heels close together for 30 seconds or longer.

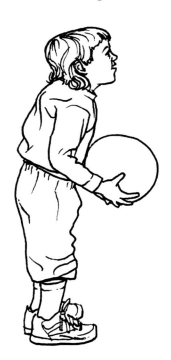

2. Step forward standing

Challenge the child to make a big step forward and then to "freeze" in place. Ask the child to stand and balance for five counts, 10 counts, and so on.

Draw an outline of feet in the biggest step as a reference for repeated trials and to see the progress made. Practice with either foot forward.

GOAL: The child stands in the big step position for 30 seconds or longer.

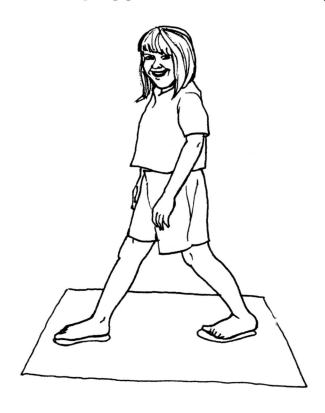

3. Standing with forefeet raised

Hold the child by the hands and ask her to stand with her forefeet on a Poly beam. (Two books may be used instead of a beam.) Encourage the child to relax, drop her heels to the floor, and try to balance independently. Count how long the child is able to balance in this position. Have her blow a whistle for entertainment.

GOAL: The child stands and balances with most of her weight over her heels for 30 seconds or longer.

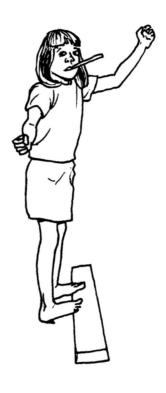

Half-Standing With Arm Support at a Table

PURPOSE: The child learns to stand and balance with most of his weight over one leg. Half-standing trains balance and control needed for single leg standing.

PRACTICE SETUP: Have the child stand with one foot on the floor and the other foot on a book, box, or bench. His feet should be flat and slightly turned out, and his flexed knee should point forward or slightly out. The higher the foot is placed, the more difficult the activity. Practice each activity first with a 4″ step-up and increase the height as the child's balance improves.

1. Half-standing at furniture

Have the child half-stand and play at a table with his favorite toys. Monitor the child's legs. The flexed knee should not turn in. Guard or assist the child as needed. Withdraw all support as the child relaxes and gains balance. Practice with either foot up.

GOAL: The child independently half-stands at a table for 2 minutes on either leg.

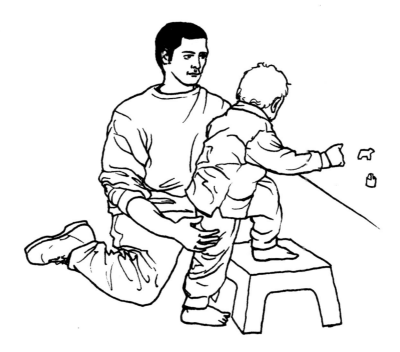

2. Half-standing with knee bend or reach

Practice as in the previous activity. Play with the child and challenge him to:

a) Bend down and reach for a toy; or
b) Reach up high for a toy.

Guard the child well, practice with either foot up, and have the child reach with either hand.

GOAL: The child half-stands independently at a table and bends down or reaches up.

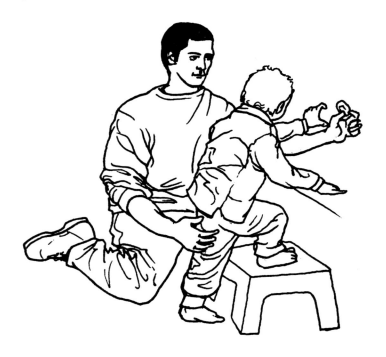

Half-Standing With
Arm Support and Assistance

PURPOSE: The child learns to stand and balance with most of his weight over one leg. Half-standing trains balance and control needed for single leg standing.

PRACTICE SETUP: The child stands with one foot on the floor and the other foot on a book, box, or bench. The feet should be flat and slightly turned out, and the flexed knee pointed forward or slightly out. The higher the foot is placed, the more difficult the activity. Practice each activity first with a 4″ step-up and increase the height as the child's balance improves

ACTIVITY: Chair-sit with your legs apart. Have the child stand between your legs, facing you. Have the child play with a simple puzzle. First:

a) Allow the child to hold onto you for support;
b) Support the bent knee with your hand; or
c) Brace the straight leg with your leg.

As the child relaxes and concentrates on play, decrease support. Encourage the child to play quietly and balance for several minutes. Practice with either leg up.

GOAL: The child plays in the half-standing position, with minimal arm support, for several minutes.

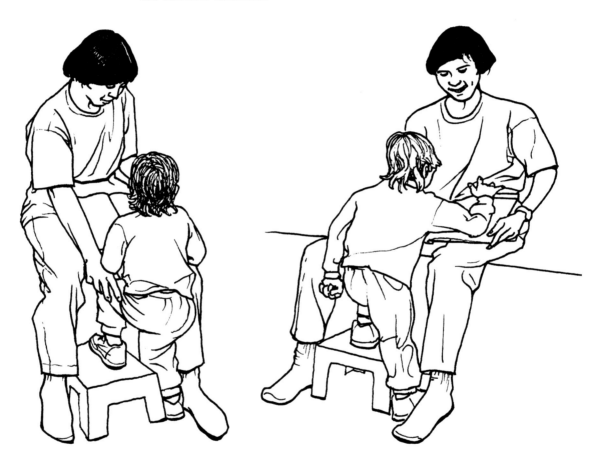

Half-Standing With Arm Support at a Wall

PURPOSE: The child learns to stand and balance with most of his weight over one leg. Half-standing trains balance and control needed for single leg standing.

PRACTICE SETUP: Have the child stand with one foot on the floor and the other foot on a book, box, or bench. His feet should be flat and slightly turned out, and his flexed leg pointed forward or slightly out. The higher the foot is placed, the more difficult the activity. Practice each activity first with a 4″ step-up and increase the height as the child's balance improves.

ACTIVITY: Have the child play in half-standing position with a dartboard on the wall, with shaving cream on a mirror or glass door, or with magnets on a refrigerator. Encourage the child to:

a) Play quietly in front;
b) Reach up high; and
c) Reach low and bend his standing leg.

Monitor the child's legs. The feet or flexed knee should not turn in. Guard or assist the child as needed. Withdraw all support as the child relaxes and gains confidence. Practice with either foot up.

GOAL: The child half-stands independently at a wall or other surface and plays for several minutes.

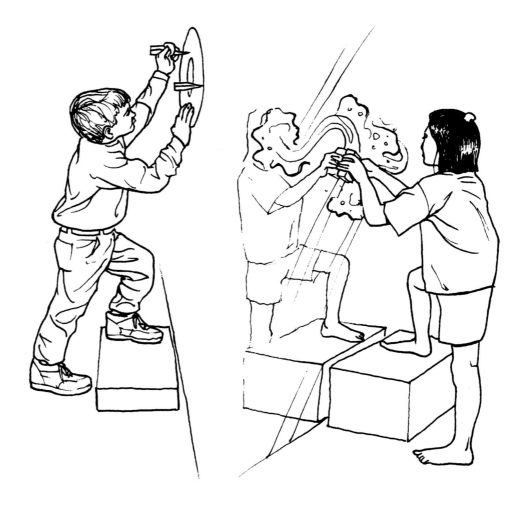

Half-Standing With Leg Support

PURPOSE: The child learns to stand and balance with most of his weight over one leg. Half-standing trains balance and control needed for single leg standing.

PRACTICE SETUP: Have the child stand with one foot flat and lightly turned out on the floor and the other foot on a knee-high bench. Assist the child by placing one hand on his bent knee and giving downward pressure. Steady the child's hip with your other hand.

1. Half-standing with leg and hip support

Start with the child bracing himself with his hands on the bench. Ask the child to raise to the standing position and balance. Challenge the child to stay for five counts, then 10 counts, and so on. Ask the child to lower his trunk and brace himself with his arms between balancing. Practice with either leg up.

GOAL: The child half-stands, with leg support, for 30 seconds or longer.

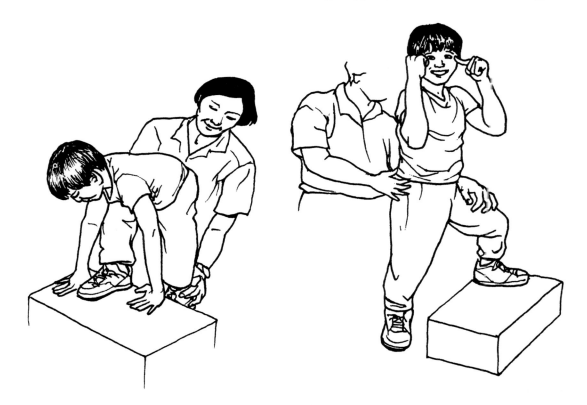

2. Half-standing with minimal leg support

The child half-stands with support to his knee and hip. As the child balances well:

a) Withdraw your support to his hip and challenge the child to balance for five, 10, 20 counts, or longer.

b) Slowly withdraw your support from his knee and challenge the child to balance for five, 10, 20 counts, or longer without any support. Practice with either leg up.

GOAL: The child half-stands with no, or minimal support, for 30 seconds or longer.

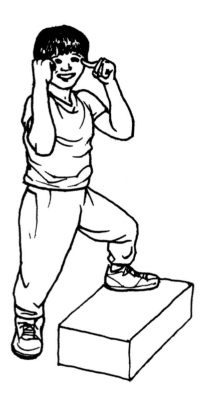

Half-Standing Without Arm Support

PURPOSE: The child learns to stand and balance with most of his weight over one leg. Half-standing trains balance and control needed for single leg standing.

PRACTICE SETUP: Have the child stand with one foot on the floor and the other foot on a book, box, or bench. His feet should be flat and slightly turned out, and his flexed knee pointed forward or slightly out. The higher the foot is placed, the more difficult the activity. Practice each activity first with a 4″ step-up and increase the height as the child's balance improves.

ACTIVITY: Chair-sit with your legs apart. Have the child stand between your legs, facing you. Choose a simple toy and play with the child. Have the child balance without any support. As the child relaxes and concentrates on play, encourage the child to:

a) Bend down and reach; or
b) Reach up high.

Guard the child well and assist if needed. Play for several minutes. Practice with either leg up and have the child reach with either hand.

GOAL: The child plays in half-standing without any support for several minutes.

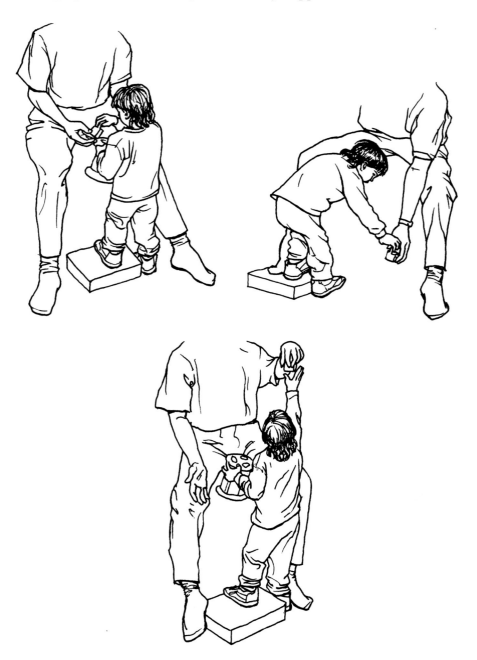

Independent Half-Standing

PURPOSE: The child learns to stand and balance with most of his weight over one leg. Half-standing trains balance and control needed for single leg standing.

PRACTICE SETUP: Have the child stand with one foot on the floor and the other foot on a book, box, or bench. His feet should be flat and slightly turned out, and his flexed knee pointed forward or slightly out. The higher the foot is placed, the more difficult the activity. Practice each activity first with a 4″ step-up and increase the height as the child's balance improves.

1. Half-standing close to the wall

Have the child half-stand with his arm supported by the wall. Once the child has gained good balance, challenge him to take his hands off the wall and stand free for five counts, then 10 counts, and so on. Practice with either leg up.

GOAL: The child half-stands independently for 30 seconds or longer.

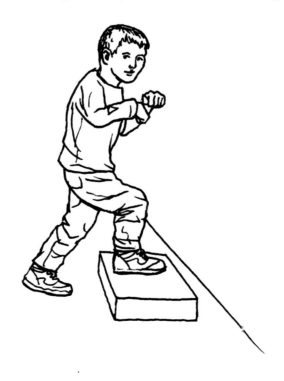

2. Half-standing in the middle of the room

Ask the child to half-stand in the middle of the room. Guard or assist the child as needed. Challenge her to balance for five counts, 10 counts, and so on. Practice with either leg up.

GOAL: The child half-stands in the middle of the room for 30 seconds or longer.

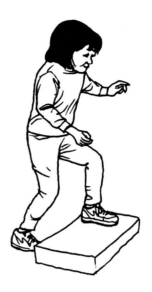

3. Half-stand with play

The child half-stands independently with good balance. Challenge her to shoot a basket. Guard the child well from the side. Practice with either leg up. This activity encourages the best upright trunk posture during independent half-standing.

GOAL: The child half-stands independently with good posture.

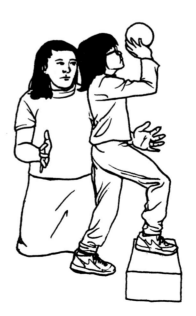

4. Half-stand with mobile step-up

Ask the child to half-stand with one foot placed on a Physio-Roll. This is a challenging activity, especially if you ask the child to move the roll forward and backward with her foot. Practice with either leg up.

GOAL: The child half-stands with one foot on a mobile surface.

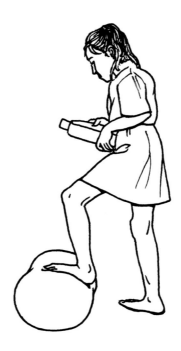

5. Advanced balance training in half-standing

Combine various activities. For instance:

a) Ask the child to swing pom-poms while half-standing;
b) Play ball with the child half-standing on a roll; and
c) Use a ball for half-standing activities.

GOAL: The child improves single leg standing balance.

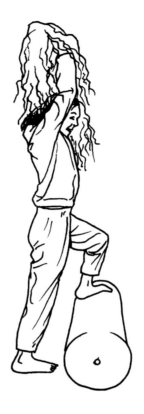 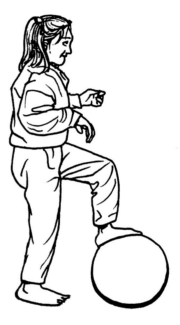

Single Leg Standing
With Arm Support

PURPOSE: These activities train single leg balance. The ability to balance on one leg is a prerequisite for important functional skills such as curb walking and stair walking.

PRACTICE SETUP: Practice in the middle of the room or as directed. The standing foot should be straight forward or slightly turned out.

1. Single leg standing with arm support

Stand facing the child and hold her hands. Ask the child to shift her weight over one foot and raise the other foot backward by bending her knee.

a) Count how long the child can stand on one foot.
b) Ask the child to do knee bends with her standing leg.

Practice with either leg.

GOAL: The child stands on one foot with hand support.

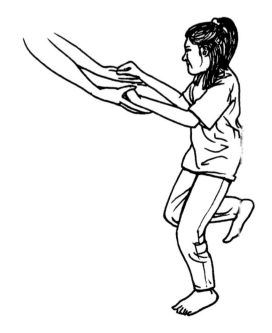

2. Single leg standing with arm support to the wall

Have the child stand with both hands against the wall. Ask her to shift her weight over one foot and lift the other foot off the floor by bending her knee and lifting her foot backward.

a) Count how long the child can balance on one foot.
b) Ask the child to do knee bends with her standing leg.

Practice with either leg.

GOAL: The child stands on one leg with arm support against the wall.

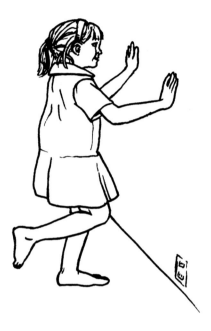

3. Single leg standing, holding onto a trapeze

Have the child hold onto a chest-high trapeze bar. Ask her to shift all her weight over one foot, steady herself, and lift her other foot off the floor. Encourage the child to:

a) Balance quietly for 30 seconds;
b) Reduce support and place only her index fingers on the bar; and
c) Do 10 knee bends with her standing leg.

Practice with either leg.

GOAL: The child single leg stands with reduced support for increasingly longer periods.

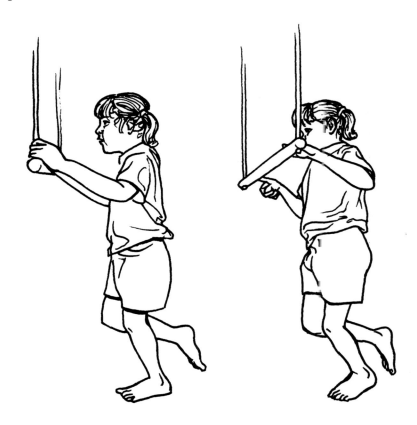

4. Single leg standing with one hand support against the wall

Ask the child to support herself with her left hand against the wall, shift all her weight over to her left leg, and raise her right foot. Once the child balances well, challenge her to reduce hand support and steady herself with one finger only. Ask the child to stand for two counts, three counts, and so on. Practice with either leg.

GOAL: The child balances for six counts with one finger against the wall.

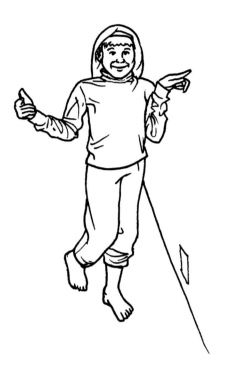

Independent Single Leg Standing

PURPOSE: These activities train single leg balance. The ability to balance on one leg is a prerequisite for important functional skills like curb walking and stair walking.

PRACTICE SETUP: Practice in the middle of the room or as directed. The standing foot should be straight forward or slightly turned out.

1. Brief single leg standing with reach

Have the child half-stand with her right foot on a 4" platform. Hold a bead, sticker, or toy high up, just out of the child's reach on the right side. Encourage the child to get it. As the child shifts her body to the right side, stretches, and reaches, her left foot will momentarily raise off the floor. Do numerous repetitions. Practice on either foot.

GOAL: The child single leg stands for brief periods.

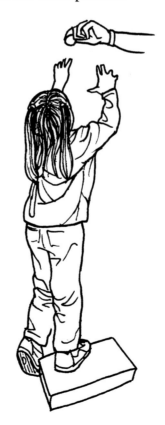

2. Single leg standing with one leg to the side

Practice single leg standing by asking the child to lift one leg to the side. This way it is easier for the child with cerebral palsy to compensate for weak hip abductor muscles. Count how long the child balances on one foot. Practice with either leg. After the child can balance with one leg lifted to the side, start practicing with one leg raised backward.

GOAL: The child single leg stands independently for brief periods.

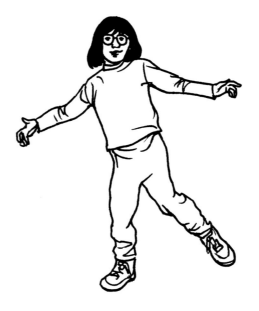

Single Leg Standing With Play

PURPOSE: These activities train single leg balance.

PRACTICE SETUP: Practice first with the child standing with her back against or close to a wall. As the child improves, practice in the middle of a carpeted room or on an Airex mat. Monitor the standing leg; that foot should be straight forward or slightly turned out.

1. Single leg standing with play

Place a beanbag on top of the child's foot; ask the child to lift it and to drop it into a container. The higher the container, the more difficult the task. Do numerous repetitions. Practice with either foot. For an additional challenge, use a penny instead of a beanbag.

GOAL: The child single leg stands with improved coordination and endurance.

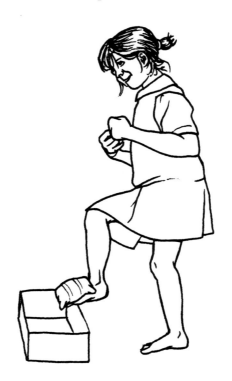

2. Single leg standing with toe grasp

Place small items on the floor and challenge the child to grasp one with her toes, lift it, and get it with the opposite hand. You may also ask the child to drop a toy into your outstretched hand or into a basket. Choose easy-to-grasp items like an eraser top, marble, bead, marker top, or small plastic toy. If the child cannot grasp with her toes, stick the item between her toes and let the child bring it up this way.

GOAL: The child single leg stands with improved coordination and endurance.

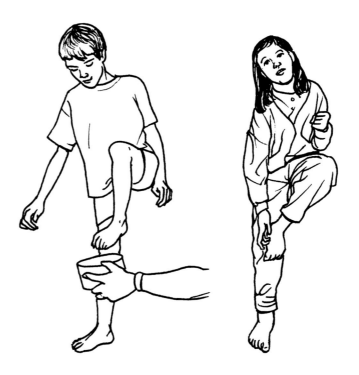

3. Other challenging activities
The child single leg stands and:

- Moves her arms;
- Swings pom-poms;
- Does knee bends; and
- Comes up on her toes.

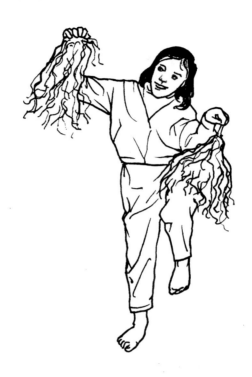

Balancing on Unstable Ground

PURPOSE: When standing on unstable ground, children need to make an extra effort to stay upright. With practice, children learn to compensate for exaggerated weight shifts caused by a foam surface. Improvement will mean better standing balance.

PRACTICE SETUP: Practice with a dense foam square. Monitor the child's foot placement. Feet should not be turned in.

1. Standing on foam

Have the child hold your hands, step onto the foam square, and stand with his feet apart and slightly turned out. Challenge the child to let go of your hands and stand independently for 10 counts, 15 counts, and so on.

GOAL: The child balances on the foam for 30 seconds or longer.

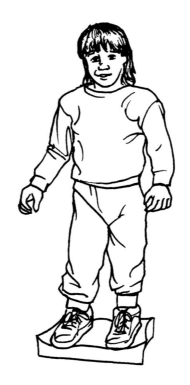

2. Standing on foam with play

Have the child stand on the foam with his feet apart and slightly turned out. Play ball with the child. Challenge him to catch and throw a ball without stepping off the foam.

GOAL: The child stands on the foam and plays ball without a loss of balance.

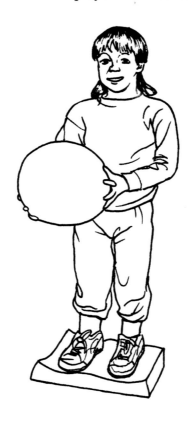

3. Step forward standing on foam

Use two foam squares. Have the child stand with each foot on a square in a step-forward position. The bigger the step, the farther the front foot is from the back one, and the more difficult the exercise. See how long the child can balance in this position. Next, challenge the child to stay in place and play ball with you. Count how many catches or throws the child can make without moving her feet. Practice with the right or left foot forward.

GOAL: The child balances in the step-forward position on the foam.

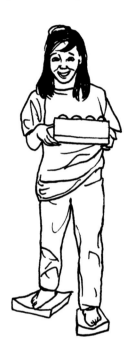

Weight Shift Training With a Balance Board

PURPOSE: These activities train side-to-side and forward and backward weight shifts. Improvement will mean better standing balance.

PRACTICE SETUP: A round balance board is used for these activities. Start with arm support. A small child may want to hold your hand. An older child may hold onto the door frame during initial practice. Use a gait belt if necessary.

1. Lateral weight shift on a balance board

Have the child stand on a balance board with his feet flat and apart. Ask the child to shift his weight to one side and then to the other. Play a simple tune and encourage the child to rock side-to-side with the rhythm. Initially, assist the child at the hips or hold his hands. As the child relaxes and enjoys the activity, withdraw your support. Closely guard the child.

GOAL: The child does controlled lateral weight shifts on a balance board.

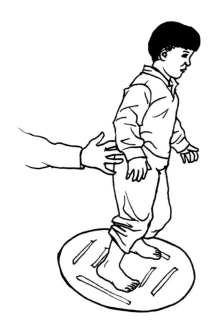

2. Forward and backward weight shift on a balance board

Have the child stand on a balance board with one foot in front and his feet flat. Ask him to shift his weight forward and then backward. Play a simple tune and encourage the child to rock forward and backward with the rhythm. Guard the child from the side. Practice with either foot forward.

GOAL: The child does controlled forward and backward weight shifts on a balance board.

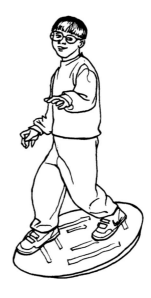

3. Circular weight shifts on a balance board

Have the child stand with his feet close together in the center of a balance board. The closer the feet, the narrower the base of support, and the more difficult the activity. Ask the child to shift his weight and tilt the board in a circular motion to the right side, then backward, to the left side, and forward. Ask the child to do 10 clockwise and 10 counterclockwise circles.

GOAL: The child does controlled small weight shifts with a narrow base of support.

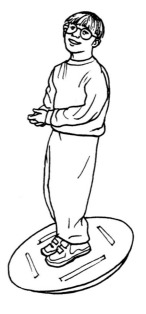

4. Squatting on a balance board

Help the child squat in the center of a balance board. After the child relaxes, withdraw your support and challenge him to balance, first with and later without arm support.

GOAL: The child squats independently on a balance board.

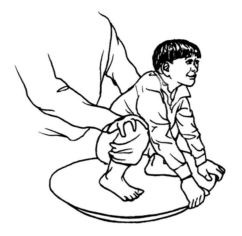

REFERENCES AND MATERIALS

1. Piper, M. C., & Darrah, J. (1994). *Motor assessment of the developing infant.* Philadelphia: W. B. Saunders.
2. Urias Pressure Splints, developed by Margaret Johnstone, available through Preston or other vendors.
3. Bottoms-Up Seat, available through Flaghouse or other vendors.
4. Bablich, K., Sochaniwskyj, A., & Koheil, R. (1986). Positional and electromyographic investigation of sitting posture of children with cerebral palsy. *Developmental Medicine and Child Neurology, 28*(5). Suppl. 53, 25.
5. Miedaner, J. A. (1990). The effects of sitting position on trunk extension for children with motor impairment. *Pediatric Physical Therapy 2*(1),11–14.
6. McClenaghan, B. A., Thombs, L., & Milner, M. (1992). Effects of seat surface inclination on postural stability and function of the upper extremities of children with cerebral palsy. *Develpmental Medicine and Child Neurology, 34,* 40–40.
7. Tilted Bench. Manufactured by Kaye Products, Inc., 535 Dimmocks Mill Road, Hillsborough, NC 27278 or The Able Generation, Inc., 1465 Woodbury Avenue, Portsmouth, NH 03801.
8. Nylatex strap. Chattanooga Corporation, 101 Memorial Drive, Box 4287, Chattanooga, TN 37405.
9. Kaye Posture System. Kaye Products, Inc., 535 Dimmocks Mill Road, Hillsborough, NC 27278.
10. Ladder of Conductive Education Set. Available through Flaghouse, Inc., 601 Flaghouse Drive, Halsbrouck Heights, NY 07604.
11. Ladderbox. Wooden box measuring 12" L x 12" W x 7" H with 46" long extentions to increase stability and 22" H ladder extending off one side. Ladder rungs are 4½" apart. Ladderbox is illustrated on page 29.
12. Airex rehab mat. Closed-cell foam mat. Available through Preston, Flaghouse, or other vendors.